EMQs for the MRCOG

John Duthie and Paul Hodges

EMQs for the MRCOG

A Guide to the Extended Matching Questions
for the MRCOG Part 2 Examination

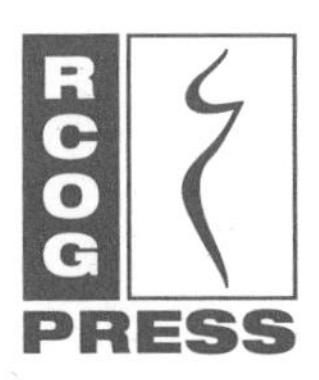

First published 2006

Product liability: Drugs and their doses are mentioned in this text. While every effort has been made to ensure the accuracy of the information contained within this publication, neither the authors nor the publishers can accept liability for errors or omissions. The final responsibility for delivery of the correct dose remains with the physician prescribing and administering the drug. In every individual case the respective user must check current indications and accuracy by consulting other pharmaceutical literature and following the guidelines laid down by the manufacturers of specific products and the relevant authorities in the country in which they are practising.

ISBN 1-904752-27-6

Published by the RCOG Press
at the Royal College of Obstetricians
and Gynaecologists
27 Sussex Place, Regent's Park
London NW1 4RG

Registered Charity No. 213280

RCOG Press Editor Jane Moody

Indexing by Liza Furnival

Text designed & typeset at the Typographic Design Unit

Printed in the United Kingdom by
Latimer Trend & Co. Ltd

Contents

Preface

The written paper for the Part 2 MRCOG examination is undergoing significant change. Extended matching questions (EMQs) are being introduced as a component of the written paper from September 2006 onwards. The purpose of the change is to develop a format of testing which probes a candidate's understanding of the subject, enables adequate coverage of the syllabus and increases the objectivity of marking.

Both of us have served on the Part 2 EMQ Sub-committee of the Royal College of Obstetricians and Gynaecologists from its foundation, working with colleagues in order to develop, discuss, debate and refine EMQs for the Part 2 examination. We have written this book to assist doctors in their preparation for success in an examination that is designed to measure their medical ability to help women. We trust that you will find our book helpful and we wish you every success in your chosen career.

John Duthie and Paul Hodges

Acknowledgements

We would like to thank Dr Michael Murphy, Director of Education, Royal College of Obstetricians and Gynaecologists, for his inspiration, unerring guidance and advice during the writing and publishing of this book.

We would also like to thank Professor Sabaratnam Arulkumaran, Vice President of the College, for his leadership in education and for writing the foreword to this book.

Thanks are also due to Wendy Reid and Ian Ramsay, respectively the founding chair and the current chair of the Part 2 EMQ Sub-committee, and all the past and present members of that Committee. Without the leadership and commitment of the chairs and the collective hard work of the Committee, the entire examination would not be in place.

Abbreviations

αFP	alphafetoprotein
βhCG	beta human chorionic gonadotrophin
ACTH	adrenocorticotrophic hormone
BMI	body mass index
CIN	cervical intraepithelial neoplasia
CMV	cytomegalovirus
CT	computed tomography
ECG	electrocardiogram
EMQ	extended matching question
FSH	follicle-stimulating hormone
Hb	haemoglobin
IgA	immunoglobulin A
IgE	immunoglobulin E
IgM	immunoglobulin M
LH	luteinising hormone
LLETZ	large-loop excision of the transformation zone
MCQ	multiple choice question
MRCOG	Membership of the Royal College of Obstetricians and Gynaecologists
MRSA	methicillin-resistant *Staphyloccus aureus*
MSU	midstream urine
PCR	polymerase chain reaction

Foreword

Education and training is at the forefront of the College's agenda. The curriculum is continuously updated and is highly fit for purpose. The clinician is expected to possess the best knowledge, clinical skills, attitude and an ability to communicate well. Patients expect treatment that is prompt, appropriate and optimal. It is the College's role to make sure that the assessment processes in place throughout training and afterwards are robust and geared to test what is necessary to be a good clinician. Several in-house continuous assessment tools, including multiprofessional feedback, have become the norm.

The examination needs to judge that the clinician is doing what is expected of them in the clinical setting. The MRCOG Part 2 examination is part of the assessment. Multiple choice questions (MCQs) and short essay questions have been used until now and will continue to be part of the examination in the future. They test knowledge in different ways. Extended matching questions (EMQs) are being introduced from September 2006. These will take this examination beyond factual recall and should test and identify a 'judgement-safe clinician'. The questions will reward reasoning as well as factual recall. EMQs will test reactions to a clinical situation, as many questions will be related to a theme and many tasks will be to derive the diagnosis and appropriate management. They will reduce ambiguity by requesting the 'most likely answer' rather than 'true or false'. EMQs allow broader clinical sampling compared with short-answer questions. Results will be more valid compared with MCQs, without sacrificing reliability. One has to accept that the examination is a stressful experience. The more one prepares, the less stressful it will be and the easier to pass. EMQs should be good news for the practicing clinician.

On behalf of the College, I would like to thank the authors, John Duthie and Paul Hodges, for producing this excellent book. They have a mix of experience as a clinician and in examining and assessment research. Both have been at the forefront of revitalising the process of the MRCOG Part 2 examination. I am sure that this book will prove to be an essential tool to prepare for the MRCOG Part 2 examination. The introduction and overall style make it easy to read and to understand. Those who are preparing for the examination, as well as clinicians practising obstetrics and gynaecology, will find this book useful.

Professor S Arulkumaran, Vice President – Education
Royal College of Obstetricians and Gynaecologists

How to use this book

The first two chapters provide some background and an introduction to the new format and will help you to decide how best to approach this examination. The next chapter, Chapter 3, provides worked examples of specimen EMQs with answers and a brief explanation. In total, there are 15 lists of options and 62 twigs (over one paper's worth). There is also some advice on how to tackle each EMQ and how to avoid mistakes.

Chapter 4 is composed of EMQs printed without answers. There are 16 lists of options, producing a total of 40 items. This particular chapter is an example of exactly what candidates will face in the written paper of the Part 2 examination leading to Membership of the Royal College of Obstetricians and Gynaecologists. To make it an exact replica of the examination to be faced, you should recreate examination conditions as best as you can (at the very least, make sure you cannot be disturbed at all) and time yourself tackling it – under an hour should be your target. Many, but not all, of the option lists will be familiar from the worked examples – however, all of the twigs are different.

Chapter 5 is another mock paper. There are ten option lists, again producing a total of 40 questions. This is totally fresh. The option lists from the worked examples are not included (six option lists which were used new for the first mock paper are repeated but again have fresh twigs). This paper should provide you with an even more realistic trial of what the new EMQ Part 2 paper will be like.

The answers to both the 'mock' papers of EMQs with 40 items each are given in Chapters 6 and 7. For the first mock paper in Chapter 6, there are references back to the relevant worked examples with the answers, where this is applicable for the first 20 questions.

Appendix 1 provides filled-in answer keys to the mock examinations. This will allow you to easily tally your:

☑ number of correct answers/40

☒ number of incorrect answers/40.

When reviewing your performance in the mock examinations, it is a good idea to make quite detailed notes on the option lists and questions that you answered incorrectly to guide your future revision.

Also included at the back of the book is a fold-out blank answer sheet (Appendix 2) for you to use when attempting the mock papers. This is only section of the book not subject to copyright. Please photocopy the sheet for easier and repeated use.

1 | The educational and evaluative benefits of EMQs

It is worth briefly covering the College's intentions in introducing this new paper and the educational and evaluative benefits of the EMQ format. Basic knowledge of these purposes should aid the candidate's preparation for this innovative new style of examination paper. Much more detail on the preparations made by the College committees and the ethos behind the new examination can be found in the article on which this chapter is based.[1]

There are a number of compelling reasons that promoted the introduction of EMQs for the College. They:

- ☑ are relatively easy to write well
- ☑ can be computer marked with unerring accuracy
- ☑ are a form of examination that will increase the validity and reliability of our overall assessment of candidates
- ☑ test more complex understanding than multiple choice questions (MCQs)
- ☑ allow a wider coverage of subjects and domain than the short answer papers.

EMQs are now widely and successfully used in undergraduate-level medical examinations and have started to be used at postgraduate level. The Royal College of Psychiatrists introduced EMQs in the Spring 2003 sitting of the Part 1 MRCPsych examination, following encouraging results in a pilot paper. They have been successfully used in the membership examinations of the Royal College of Surgeons (Glasgow and London) and Royal College of General Practitioners. Also, the Royal College of Paediatrics and Child Health uses EMQs in its Diploma in Child Health. The PLAB test is entirely in EMQ format. They are also clearly more objective than the short answer (essay type) questions. The short answers require candidates to surmise exactly what is required of them and what the examiner will reward. As a result, they probably do not assess medical reasoning as well as would be hoped, or as one review article phrases it: 'Their format is commonly believed to be intrinsically superior to a multiple choice format. Much evidence shows, however, that this assumed superiority is limited'.[2] They also require the candidate to write in well-constructed English – something that candidates whose first language is not English may not find easy.[3] Moreover, educational research clearly indicates that examinations, particularly those with a high stake such as the Part 2 MRCOG, are improved by increasing the number of performance indicators through increasing the number of test formats.[4]

EMQs will drive the learning required to pass the Part 2 MRCOG in slightly different ways than the two current questions formats. The MCQs tend to require a rather rote memorising of facts and figures. For the short answers, candidates tend to revise a rather limited range of topics, whether current 'hot' topics or predictable areas of discussion. EMQs require good knowledge across the broad range of obstetric and gynaecological practice. Good clinical knowledge will be the key, particularly applied clinical knowledge. It is clear that the domains of management, diagnosis and investigation will be the most frequently tested and these will be the most important areas for revision.

Perhaps the most important message, though, is not to worry too much. EMQs, after all, will currently only contribute 15% of your overall mark in the Part 2 written examination.

REFERENCES

1. Duthie SJ, Hodges PD, Ramsay IN, Reid WMN. Extended Matching Questions: a new component of the Part 2 examination leading to Membership of the Royal College of Obstetricians and Gynaecologists. *The Obstetrician & Gynaecologist* 2006; **8**: 181–5.

2. Schuwirth LWT, van der Vleuten CPM. Written assessment. *BMJ* 2003; **326**: 643–5.

3. Stobart G. Fairness in multicultural assessment systems. *Assessment in Education* 2005; **12**: 275–87.

4. Linn RL. Assessments and accountability. *Educational Researcher* 2000; **29**, 2: 4–12.

2 | EMQ answering technique

Introduction

A candidate with a sound knowledge of obstetrics and gynaecology who has received the appropriate supervised training and gained adequate clinical experience should have little difficulty in tackling EMQs. However, failure to appreciate the relationship between knowledge and technique may affect your performance in the examination. Essentially, both your knowledge and technique should be sound.

The overall purpose of the EMQ is to probe a candidate's understanding of clinical obstetrics and gynaecology. They tend to assess the application of medical knowledge rather than simple recall, by giving a number of possible answers to a short clinical problem. They are replacing a number of the true/false multiple-choice questions (MCQs) and slightly reducing the need to write short answer questions (essays), which would be marked by subject matter experts.

Attributes of EMQs

So what are the main differences between EMQs and these more familiar types of formats for assessment?

With the wider number of options available, it is obvious that the educated guess becomes a far less valuable technique than in the 50:50 world of the true or false MCQ. Studies demonstrate that even in negatively marked MCQ papers all candidates should benefit substantially from backing their educated guesses and only a small percentage lose marks by backing their wild guesses.[1] The RCOG MCQ and EMQ papers are not negatively marked, making the technique potentially even more potent.

That does not mean that an educated guess is not sometimes appropriate for EMQs. The popular and renowned advice to go with the first answer you think of first seems to be gaining ever more support. See, for example, Malcolm Gladwell's non-fiction bestseller, *Blink: The Power of Thinking Without Thinking*.[2] Essentially, for the EMQ paper, your guessing needs to be judicious. This book therefore provides much advice on the best strategy for minimising your risk of answering incorrectly and maximising your possible score. Each worked example covers this topic. As with the true/false MCQ paper, there is no negative marking. However, even 'good guessing' may well lead to an unsustainably high number of mistakes in the EMQ paper. While EMQs do not reach the levels of synthesis of clinical knowledge that can be tested in the short answers, they do test more complex understanding than MCQs. Simple knowledge recall suffices for correctly answering many true/false MCQs. This will continue to apply to some EMQs but most will require some working through.

Solid, applied clinical knowledge will be required to answer the majority of EMQs. A number will have quite substantial clinical scenarios to interpret. In recognition of their increased length and complexity, in particular with regard to the extra time required to read them, EMQs have been assigned a longer time for completion than MCQs. It is important to bear this in mind when preparing for the examination.

Structure of EMQs

The structure of an EMQ is as follows:

- ☑ a list of options
- ☑ a lead-in statement or paragraph
- ☑ the items.

The number of options on the list will vary from a minimum of four up to a maximum of 20. There are thus 20 spaces lettered *A* to *T* to fill in on the answer sheet (see our example provided for the mock examinations at the end of this book). The majority of questions in the examination will have around 10–14 options in their lists. As far as reasonably possible, the list of options is made homogeneous; that is, most options will be broadly equivalent or at least in similar areas. The option lists will nearly always be in alphabetical or numerical order for ease of reference; if not, they will be in the most appropriate order for quick reference.

In the examination itself, each option list will then have from one to five items; that is, self-contained questions based on those options. We have provided more in our examples, to give more thorough revision.

Candidates should find this technique useful in tackling EMQs:

1. Read the lead-in statement first.
2. Ask yourself the question – 'Do I really understand what the lead-in statement says?'
3. Consider each item one by one.
4. Develop the answer to the item in your mind.
5. Finally, select the correct answer from the list of options and enter your answer into the mark sheet.

Candidates are not advised to read through the list of options first. There is a small but live possibility of being wrongly cued by distractors among the options by doing this. The lead-in statement will generally be very clear as to the task required and should leave no room for ambiguity. Reading it carefully and understanding it will be the key to performing the task required in the right manner and thus answering the question correctly. Then, for candidates with an appropriate standard of knowledge and experience, it will be a simple matter to answer the items. Consider Worked Example 1, taken from a totally different area than obstetrics and gynaecology, so there are no distractions.

WORKED EXAMPLE 1

Theme ▷ Biblical history (Genesis/Noah).

Domain ▷ Knowledge/understanding.

Options

A	2	F	6
B	2000	G	18
C	0	H	81
D	24	I	90
E	12	J	1000

The following item refers to Biblical history. Select the correct answer from the list of options.

Item 1 ▶ How many **pairs** of animals did Moses take into the boat called the Ark?
Answer ▷ C=0.

Item 2 ▶ How many **pairs** of 'unclean' animals did Noah take into the boat called the Ark?
Answer ▷ C=0.

Commentary

There are ten options, followed by a short and precise lead-in statement. There are two items and the word 'pairs' is emboldened as a distractor in each item. The answer is *C* in *Item 1*. This is because Noah, not Moses, took animals into the boat called the Ark [Genesis 5 : 1–5]. A candidate who focuses on 'pairs' and the 'Ark' may well be trying to achieve the answer by guess work. The Patriach who did take animals into the Ark is named correctly in *Item 2*. But the answer is still *C*. Why? Noah took seven of each unclean animal into the Ark. As seven is an odd number, no pairs were possible, despite the popular nursery rhyme, 'The animals went in two by two' which refers to 'clean' animals. A full reading of the item and sound knowledge of the Biblical passage in question leads to the correct answers.

Don't worry – none of the MRCOG EMQs will be this tricky!

Consider the next example, which is more straightforward but is again from a different area than obstetrics and gynaecology to avoid distraction.

WORKED EXAMPLE 2

Theme ▷ Gregorian calendar.

Domain ▷ Knowledge/application.

Options

A	0	G	6
B	1	H	7
C	2	I	9
D	3	J	10
E	4	K	11
F	5	L	12

The items listed below refer to days in the months of the Gregorian calendar. For each item, select the most appropriate number from the list of options. Each option may be used once, more than once or not at all.

Item 1 ▶ How many months have 28 days?
Answer ▷ *L*= 12.

Item 2 ▶ How many months have only 28 days?
Answer ▷ *B*= 1.

Commentary

There are 12 options and the lead-in statement is very clear and states that the items listed below refer to days in the months of the Gregorian rather than the lunar or any other type of calendar. The candidate is asked to select the most appropriate number from the list of options for each of the items. Although the wording in each item is very similar, the answers are different. An elementary knowledge of the Gregorian calendar is required, together with a careful reading of the text of each item. How many months have 28 days? The answer – 'all of them' – i.e. 12. Therefore the answer to *Item 1* is *L*= 12. However, if the wording of the question is 'how many' have only 28 days, then the answer is 1. Therefore the answer to *Item 2* is *B*. The absolute majority of candidates attempting this EMQ would get both items correct. However, a candidate with only the vaguest notion of the Gregorian calendar and who does not read the question properly is likely to fail both items.

Again, do not worry, none of the MRCOG EMQs will be aiming to deliberately mislead like this example. However, there will be distractors, particularly in the option lists.

More option list examples

The EMQs for the Part 2 MRCOG examination will contain many different lists of options. The following are examples of the sorts of lists that will be used:

- ☑ Options for management
- ☑ Patient profiles
- ☑ Tumour profiles
- ☑ Obstetric conditions
- ☑ Gynaecological conditions
- ☑ Advice given to women
- ☑ Levels of risk
- ☑ Complications
- ☑ Different types of obstetric operations
- ☑ Different types of gynaecological operations
- ☑ Lists of investigations
- ☑ Results of investigations
- ☑ Results of screening tests
- ☑ Endocrine profiles
- ☑ Different anatomical structures
- ☑ Results of postmortem examinations.

Pass marks

Unfortunately, it is too early to know what sort of pass marks will be set for the EMQ paper. These will, of course, vary owing to standard setting. However, as guesswork plays a far lower role in EMQs than MCQs it is almost inconceivable that the high pass marks of the true/false MCQ paper (generally in the region of 78–82%) will be duplicated. A pass mark of somewhere between 55% and 70% is almost certain, with the region of 62–67% a good bet.

REFERENCES

1. Hammond EJ, McIncloe AK, Sansome AJ, Spargo PM. Multipe-choice examinations: adopting an evidence-based approach to exam technique. *Anaesthesia* 1998; **53**: 1105–8.

2. Gladwell M. *Blink: The Power of Thinking Without Thinking*. New York: Little Brown and Company; 2005.

3 | Worked examples

STEM/OPTION LIST 1

Theme ▷ Obstetrics: perinatal mortality rate.

Domain ▷ Epidemiology, statistics.

Options

A	10	I	10 000
B	100	J	10 880
C	120	K	12 880
D	200	L	19 000
E	250	M	19 100
F	500	N	19 500
G	1000	O	19 880
H	2000	P	1 80

Instructions

In a certain region, all pregnant women booked for antenatal care and all gestations were reliably measured, and all late fetal losses were notified and registered. The perinatal mortality rate was 10/1000 total births and there were 100 late fetal losses and 80 first-week neonatal deaths. During the time that the perinatal mortality rate was measured, there were 20 000 total births. For each of the items listed below, select the **single** correct number from the list of options. Each option may be used once, more than once or not at all.

Item 1 ▶ What was the number of stillbirths?
Answer ▷ *C*= 120.

Item 2 ▶ What was the number of perinatal deaths?
Answer ▷ *D*= 200.

Item 3 ▶ What was the number of live births?
Answer ▷ *O*= 19 880.

Commentary

Purpose

The purpose of this question is to test your understanding of the meaning of 'the perinatal mortality rate'.

Content

In this question, the list of options comprises a set of numbers. The numbers range from '10' to '19 980'. As in all the extended matching questions the lead-in statement is very important. Following the lead-in statement there are three questions or 'items'. You are expected to read the lead-in statement, examine each item and work out the answer before selecting the answer from the list of options.

The lead-in statement leaves no room for ambiguity. All the information that you require is contained within the lead-in statement and a candidate with a good understanding of the term 'perinatal mortality rate' would find the questions that follow very easy.

Answers

The perinatal mortality rate was 10/1000 total births. Therefore, in 20 000 total births the total number of perinatal deaths was comprised as follows:

1. 120 stillbirths.
2. 80 first-week neonatal deaths (as stated in the lead-in statement).

Therefore, the answer to *Item 1* is *C* and the answer to *Item 2* is *D*.

As there were 20 000 births in total, with 120 stillbirths, then the number of live births was 20 000 minus 120, which equals 19 880.

Therefore, the answer to *Item 3* is *O*.

Minimising the risk and maximising your score

Read the question carefully. This particular example serves to illustrate how simple and straightforward an EMQ is designed to be. Candidates who do not understand the 'perinatal mortality rate' are at risk of guessing and selecting incorrect answers. If you do understand the subject you would be able to work out the answers to the three items without the use of a calculator and within a very short space of time.

This example also illustrates one of the major pitfalls. Be very wary of getting mixed up with numbers. Under the stressful conditions of an examination it is understandable that a candidate misreads numbers. If the perinatal mortality rate is 10/1000 total births and there are 20 000 births, then the total number of perinatal deaths (including stillbirths and first-week neonatal deaths) is 200. The list of options in this particular EMQ is relatively long and there are several 'distractors' present. For example, '19 880' and '19 980' look very similar. You must not be distracted by the presence of the number '10' as 'option *A*'. The perinatal mortality rate is 10/1000 total births and option A is not an answer to any of the items. The number of late fetal losses has no bearing on the answers to the items. The statement 'and there were 100 late fetal losses' is merely a distractor. The candidate who knows that the perinatal mortality rate comprises the number of stillbirths and first-week neonatal deaths per 1000 total births would have little difficulty in obtaining full marks for this EMQ.

STEM/OPTION LIST 2

Theme ▷ Obstetrics and gynaecology: drug usage, mode of administration.

Domain ▷ Management.

Options

A Bladder irrigation
B Bolus subcutaneous injection; repeated
C Bolus subcutaneous injection; stat
D Continuous intravenous infusion
E Continuous subcutaneous infusion
F Implant
G Inhalation of a nebulised spray
H Intramuscular
I Intrathecal

J Intravenous injection
K Nasal drops
L Per oram
M Per vaginam
N Retention enema
O Sublingual
P Topical application
Q Via central venous line
R Via nasogastric tube

Instructions

The following scenarios refer to women who require treatment or palliation for various conditions. Select the **single** most appropriate route of administration for the pharmacological agent that is to be used from the list of options. Each option may be used once, more than once or not at all.

Item 1 ▶ A woman is undergoing abdominal hysterectomy for a benign condition and has been given an intravenous injection of amoxicillin trihydrate and potassium clavulanate. An acute anaphylactic reaction develops and **adrenaline** needs to be given.
Answer ▷ *H* = Intramuscular.

Item 2 ▶ A pregnant woman develops idiopathic preterm labour at a gestation of 28 weeks. After appropriate assessment it is decided that **betamethasone** must be given.
Answer ▷ *H* = Intramuscular.

Item 3 ▶ A pregnant woman in labour with ruptured membranes has been given intravenous oxytocin for the augmentation of labour. Uterine hypersystole occurs with a non-reassuring cardiotocogram. Following appropriate assessment and counselling, a decision is taken to carry out emergency caesarean section. However, the operating theatre is occupied and a decision is taken to administer **terbutaline**.
Answer ▷ *D* = Continuous intravenous infusion.

Item 4 ▶ A woman is undergoing cytotoxic chemotherapy for choriocarcinoma in the appropriate centre. As part of the regimen **vincristine** needs to be given.
Answer ▷ *D*=Continuous intravenous infusion.

Item 5 ▶ A woman is undergoing cytotoxic chemotherapy for ovarian cancer in the appropriate centre. As part of the regimen, **carboplatin** needs to be given.
Answer ▷ *D*=Continuous intravenous infusion.

Commentary

Content

This EMQ contains a relatively long list of 18 options. The lead-in statement is suitably short but precise. The candidate is asked to consider different clinical scenarios where women must receive treatment or palliation for various conditions. The candidate is asked to select the most appropriate route of administration of a certain drug from the list of options. Again, there is the standard statement that 'each option may be used once, more than once or not at all'.

Answers

Item 1=H ▶ The first choice for the route of administration of adrenaline in the case of anaphylactic shock is intramuscular.

Item 2=H ▶ Steroids in preterm labour are given as an intramuscular injection.

Item 3=D ▶ In this situation, terbutaline is given as a continuous intravenous infusion.

Item 4=D ▶ Vincristine is to be used as a continuous intravenous infusion.

Item 5=D ▶ Carboplatin is given as a continuous intravenous infusion.

Minimising risk and maximising your score

This is a straightforward question, which tests the application of clinical knowledge. The EMQ merely asks the candidate to choose an appropriate method of administration. There is no need to justify the use of a certain drug in a certain situation or to consider better alternatives. The answers to each item are obvious and can be easily selected from the list of options. This is a prime example of an EMQ where the importance of reading the lead-in statement, then reading the item, having a mental picture of the answer and choosing it quickly from the list is illustrated. Candidates could easily and dangerously waste time assessing and weighing up the long list of options for each question asked. Candidates with good examination technique can build up a highly useful bank of additional time by maintaining a good pace through questions like these.

STEM/OPTION LIST 3

Theme ▷ Obstetrics: prevalence study on gestational diabetes mellitus.

Domain ▷ Research/statistics.

Options

Prevalence study on gestational diabetes mellitus:

	Null hypothesis	
	TRUE	FALSE
No statistically significant difference	A	B
Statistically significant difference leading to rejection of the null hypothesis	C	D

Instructions

A research team conducts a study to investigate the prevalence of gestational diabetes mellitus in two cities: one in Asia and the other in Europe. After the appropriate data are collected, the researchers carry out statistical tests with various levels of power and draw their conclusions. The items below refer to various possible conclusions apropos the null hypothesis. The table above, containing the list of options, shows different conclusions. For each item, select the **single** option which describes the conclusion of the researchers. Each option may be used once, more than once or not at all.

Item 1 ▶ The null hypothesis is true and it is accepted by the researchers that there is no statistically significant difference between the two populations.
Answer ▷ *A* = No statistically significant difference. Null hypothesis: TRUE.

Item 2 ▶ There is a statistically significant difference in the prevalence of gestational diabetes mellitus between the two populations and on this basis the researchers reject the null hypothesis when it is actually true.
Answer ▷ *C* = Statistically significant difference leading to rejection of the null hypothesis. Null hypothesis: TRUE.

Item 3 ▶ The researchers make a type-2 error.
Answer ▷ *B* = No statistically significant difference. Null hypothesis: FALSE.

Item 4 ▶ The researchers do find a statistically significant difference between the two populations when the null hypothesis is actually false. The null hypothesis is rejected.
Answer ▷ *D* = Statistically significant difference leading to rejection of the null hypothesis. Null hypothesis: FALSE.

Commentary

Purpose

Using this EMQ, the examiners wish to assess your understanding of basic research methodology. Even after statistical analysis has been applied, can the null hypothesis be accepted or rejected incorrectly?

Content

There are only four options in the list of options and they are presented in a tabular form. The lead-in statement is relatively lengthy and describes how a research team conducts a comparative study on the prevalence of gestational diabetes mellitus. The research team studies two cities – one in Asia and the other in Europe. The appropriate data is analysed, the research team carried out statistical tests and draws conclusions. It is stated clearly that the studies used various levels of power. Each of the four items describes a different outcome of the research.

Answers

Item 1 = A ▶ The null hypothesis is that there is no difference between the two populations; as stated in *Item 1* it is actually TRUE and the null hypothesis is accepted by the researchers as there is no statistical significant difference between the two populations. Therefore, the conclusion of the research team is correct.

Item 2 = C ▶ The null hypothesis is ACTUALLY TRUE. However, the research team does find a statistically significant difference in the prevalence of gestational diabetes mellitus between the two populations. The research team makes a type-I error by rejecting the null hypothesis when it is actually true.

Item 3 = B ▶ In this scenario, the null hypothesis is ACTUALLY FALSE and there is a real difference between the two populations. However, the research team fails to identify that there is a statistically significant difference between the two populations using the data which the team collected and therefore a type-2 error has been made.

Item 4 = D ▶ The null hypothesis is ACTUALLY FALSE and it is correctly rejected.

Minimising risk and maximising your score

You need to understand the concept of the null hypothesis, how it can be incorrectly accepted or rejected, type-1 error and type-2 error. When in doubt, construct your own 4 × 4 table and work out the answers on a separate piece of paper.

STEM/OPTION LIST 4

Theme ▷ Obstetrics: maternal infection/toxoplasmosis.

Domain ▷ Diagnosis.

Options

A Acute maternal CMV with equivocal evidence of fetal infection
B Acute maternal toxocara infection
C Acute maternal toxoplasmosis
D Acute maternal toxoplasmosis infection with equivocal evidence of fetal infection
E Acute maternal toxoplasmosis infection with fetal infection
F Acute maternal toxoplasmosis infection with no fetal infection
G Acute maternal tularaemia
H Chronic maternal CMV infection
I Chronic maternal toxocara infection
J Maternal Q fever
K No evidence of maternal toxoplasmosis
L Previous maternal toxoplasmosis

Worked examples

Instructions

The following clinical scenarios refer to a pregnant woman who has previously been in good health and who has developed headache, fever, fatigue and sore throat. The outstanding clinical sign on examination is generalised lymphadenopathy. The results of various investigations are provided in the items below. For each item choose the **single** most likely diagnosis from the list of options. Each option may be used once, more than once or not at all.

Item 1 ▶ Sabin-Feldman dye test on maternal serum is positive at very high titre.
Answer ▷ *C*=Acute maternal toxoplasmosis.

Item 2 ▶ Sabin-Feldman dye test is positive at low titre and the corresponding IgM titre is positive at a very low titre. Three weeks later the tests on maternal serum are repeated and the Sabin-Feldman dye test is positive at high titre and the corresponding IgM titre is unequivocally higher than 3 weeks previously.
Answer ▷ *C*=Acute maternal toxoplasmosis.

Item 3 ▶ Sabin-Feldman dye test is positive at low titre and the corresponding IgM titre is positive at a very low titre. Three and six weeks later the tests on maternal serum are repeated and the results are the same.
Answer ▷ *L*=Previous maternal toxoplasmosis.

Item 4 ▶ Sabin-Feldman dye test is negative and the corresponding IgM, IgE, and IgA are undetectable in maternal serum.
Answer ▷ *K*=No evidence of maternal toxoplasmosis.

Item 5 ▶ Sabin-Feldman dye test is positive at high titre, the corresponding IgM titre is high in maternal serum and polymerase chain reaction carried out on a sample of amniotic fluid obtained at amniocentesis is positive for *Toxoplasma gondii*.
Answer ▷ *E*=Acute maternal toxoplasmosis infection with fetal infection.

Item 6 ▶ Sabin-Feldman dye test is positive at high titre, the corresponding IgM titre is high in maternal serum and polymerase chain reaction carried out on a sample of amniotic fluid obtained at amniocentesis is negative for *Toxoplasma gondii*.
Answer ▷ *F*=Acute maternal toxoplasmosis infection with no fetal infection.

Item 7 ▶ Sabin-Feldman dye test is positive at high titre, the corresponding IgM titre is high in maternal serum and ultrasound examination shows the presence of isolated mild ventriculomegaly.
Answer ▷ *D*=Acute maternal toxoplasmosis infection with equivocal evidence of fetal infection.

Commentary

Purpose

To probe candidates' understanding of diagnostic tests for maternal and fetal toxoplasmosis.

Content

There is a list of options comprising 12 different diagnoses, a lead-in statement and seven items. The list of options comprises infections due to various different organisms: viral, rickettsial, spirochaetal and protozoal. There are several distractors in the list of options. The lead-in statement describes a pregnant woman who has developed headache, fever, fatigue and sore throat, having previously been in good health. The clinical symptoms exclude several of the distractors. The outstanding clinical sign on examination is described as being generalised lymphadenopathy. The lead-in statement goes on to say that the results of various investigations are provided in the items and the candidates are asked to select the most likely diagnosis for each item.

Answers

In order tackle this EMQ, the candidate must possess knowledge of serology and be able to apply that knowledge in different clinical scenarios. The following knowledge is required:

1. The Sabin-Feldman dye test is a measure of immunoglobulin G (IgG) against *Toxoplasma gondii*. Organisms mixed with serum containing no antibody and methylene blue stain deeply with the blue dye. However, organisms exposed to serum that contains antibody to *T. gondii* in the presence of complement, and in the presence of methylene blue, do not stain.
2. Serological tests for IgM, IgE and IgA antibodies to *T. gondii* are also available.
3. A positive Sabin–Feldman dye test and the presence of IgM in high titre would establish a diagnosis of acute toxoplasmosis.
4. If the titres are low, it would be advisable to check the antibody levels 3 weeks apart. Serial rising titres usually confirm the presence of acute infection.
5. Reproducibility of some of the tests is problematic and best done in reference laboratories.
6. Polymerase chain reaction (PCR) testing for *T. gondii* in amniotic fluid appears to be very accurate in identifying infection of the fetus.

Most of this knowledge is fairly basic; the remainder should be picked up in a good revision regimen.

Items 1 & 2 = C

Item 3 = L ▶ In this scenario, the Sabin–Feldman dye test is positive at low titre and the corresponding IgM titre is positive but at a very low level. Serial testing shows no change and therefore, the answer is *L*.

Item 4 = K ▶ This is straightforward – there is no serological evidence of toxoplasmosis infection at the time the test was carried out. Therefore, the answer is *K*.

Item 5 = E ▶ In this scenario, there is evidence of maternal and fetal infection as the PCR test is positive for *T. gondii* when amniotic fluid obtained at amniocentesis is investigated. Therefore, the answer is *E*.

Item 6 = F ▶ In this scenario, there is evidence of acute maternal toxoplasmosis but the PCR test on amniotic fluid is negative. Therefore, the answer is *F*.

Item 7 = D ▶ In this scenario, there is evidence of acute maternal toxoplasmosis with evidence of isolated mild fetal ventriculomegaly. There is a high index of suspicion that the fetus may be infected with *T. gondii* but it is not certain, as there are other causes of ventriculomegaly. Therefore, the answer is *D*.

Minimising risk and maximising your score

This EMQ demands that candidates are able to apply their basic knowledge to clinical situations. The EMQ demonstrates the importance of reading, appropriate case discussion and thoughts on clinical management while revising for the Part 2 MRCOG examination. The long list of options may appear formidable to some candidates, as it includes some rare protozoal and spirochaetal infections. However, with a good basic knowledge of diagnostic serology as applied to *T. gondii*, there is no need to even consider several of the other options.

STEM/OPTION LIST 5

Theme ▷ Obstetrics: prepregnancy, antenatal counselling – congenital adrenal hyperplasia.

Domain ▷ Genetics.

Options

A	0	I	1 in 8
B	1 in 250	J	1 in 4
C	1 in 100	K	2 in 7
D	1 in 28	L	1 in 3
E	1 in 25	M	3 in 8
F	1 in 20	N	3 in 7
G	1 in 16	O	1 in 2
H	1 in 12	P	2 in 3

Instructions

A pregnant woman consults you for advice, as there is a family history of congenital adrenal hyperplasia. Genetic and biochemical studies show that the woman and her partner are carriers of 21-hydroxylsase deficiency. The woman has various questions, which are listed in the items. Select the **single** most appropriate answer to each question from the above list of options. Each option may be used once, more than once or not at all.

Item 1 ▶ What is the risk of an affected child in this pregnancy?
Answer ▷ *J*= 1 in 4.

Item 2 ▶ What is the risk of an affected son in this pregnancy?
Answer ▷ *I*= 1 in 8.

Item 3 ▶ What is the risk of the child being a carrier in this pregnancy?
Answer ▷ O= 1 in 2.

Item 4 ▶ If this pregnancy is affected by a child with congenital adrenal hyperplasia, what is the risk of an affected child in the next pregnancy?
Answer ▷ *J*= 1 in 4.

Commentary

Purpose

The purpose of this EMQ is to test your understanding of autosomal recessive inheritance. Are you able to give practical advice to a pregnant woman with a family history of congenital adrenal hyperplasia caused by 21-hydroxylase deficiency?

Content

The list of options comprises 16 different levels of risk, ranging from 2 in 3 to 0. The lead-in describes a pregnant woman with a family history of congenital adrenal hyperplasia due to 21-hydroxylase deficiency and it is clear that the woman and her partner are both carriers. Neither is affected – the question clearly states that they are both carriers. The lead-in statement is followed by four items which represent various questions that the pregnant woman may ask you in the antenatal clinic.

Answers

Item 1 = J ▶ The risk of an affected child is 1 in 4, therefore, the answer is *J*.

Item 2 = I ▶ The risk of an affected son is 1 in 4 × 1 in 2 = 1 in 8; therefore, the answer is *I*.

Item 3 = O ▶ Overall there is a 1 in 4 risk of an affected child, a 1 in 2 risk of a carrier child and a 1 in 4 chance that the child would neither be affected nor be a carrier, therefore, the answer is *O*.

Item 4 = J ▶ The chance of an affected child in a subsequent pregnancy is also 1 in 4, even if the present pregnancy is complicated by a child with congenital adrenal hyperplasia.

Minimising risk and maximising your score

In order to answer this question correctly, you need to be aware of the mode of inheritance of congenital adrenal hyperplasia due to 21-hydroxylase deficiently. The condition is not sex linked but pregnant women may commonly ask what the risk of an affected child of a certain sex would be. Another misconception may well be that the chances of an affected child in a subsequent pregnancy are either significantly reduced or significantly increased if the child in the present pregnancy is affected. It is also important not to get confused by numbers or by misreading the numbers.

STEM/OPTION LIST 6

Theme ▷ Obstetrics, prepregnancy, antenatal counselling.

Domain ▷ Genetics, X-linked dominant.

Options

A	0	I	1 in 3
B	1 in 100	J	4 in 10
C	1 in 88	K	1 in 2
D	1 in 25	L	2 in 3
E	1 in 16	M	3 to 1
F	1 in 8	N	2 to 1
G	1 in 4	O	3 to 2
H	3 in 10	P	1 in 1

Instructions

A man with Vitamin D-resistant rickets has three affected children. Unfortunately, his first wife, with whom he had these children, died a few years ago. He has since remarried. His new wife is a healthy woman, who is now pregnant with the man's baby and she consults you. The woman asks you various questions concerning the risks to her baby. The items refer to the woman's questions. Select the **single** most appropriate answer to the woman's questions from the list of options above. Each option may be used once, more than once or not at all.

Item 1 ▶ What is the risk of having an affected child?
Answer ▷ *K* = 1 in 2.

Item 2 ▶ What is the risk of having an affected son?
Answer ▷ *A* = 0.

Item 3 ▶ If the baby is female, what is the risk of being affected?
Answer ▷ *P* = 1 in 1.

Commentary

Purpose

To test your understanding of the mode of inheritance of an X-linked dominant condition and to test the advice you would give to a pregnant woman in the antenatal clinic.

Content

The EMQ comprises 16 options which describe various levels of risk, from 0 to 1 in 1. The lead-in statement describes a man who has vitamin D-resistant rickets and three affected children. Subsequently, the man is widowed and he then marries a healthy woman who becomes pregnant. The question makes it quite clear that the man has vitamin D-resistant rickets and the pregnant woman does not. The pregnant woman attends the antenatal clinic and requests your advice. Each of the items refers to a different question on the risk of having an affected child.

Answers

A man with vitamin D-resistant rickets who marries a healthy woman would have affected daughters and unaffected sons, therefore the answers are as follows:

Item 1 = *K*.
Item 2 = *A*.
Item 3 = *P*.

Minimising risk and maximising your score

The EMQ is very straightforward. However, it is imperative that you read the items carefully. The risk of having an affected child is 1 in 2 – all the daughters would be affected and all the sons would be unaffected. As no information is provided to the contrary, candidates should assume that this couple has an equal chance of having an offspring of either gender. Candidates may be confused by the fact that an affected man has unaffected sons. If the baby is female then the risk of being affected is 1 in 1 (*Item 3*). However, in this particular clinical scenario, the condition is carried on the X chromosome of the man. The situation would be different if the woman was affected by vitamin D-resistant rickets and the man was healthy.

STEM/OPTION LIST 7

Theme ▷ Obstetrics: labour complications, unstable lie.

Domain ▷ Management.

Options

- A Allow home
- B Apply suprapubic pressure
- C Await spontaneous labour following admission
- D Forewater amniotomy
- E Hind water amniotomy using a Drew-Smythe catheter
- F Insert prostaglandin E_2 per vaginam
- G Insert prostaglandin I_2 per vaginam
- H Lower-segment caesarean section
- I Stabilising induction of labour
- J Upper-segment caesarean section

Instructions

The clinical scenarios listed below refer to a healthy pregnant woman with three living children, all of whom were delivered normally (unless stated otherwise in the items below). She is pregnant for the fourth time. It is discovered that the lie of the fetus is unstable in the absence of placenta praevia, polyhydramnios, uterine malformation, fetal abnormality, multiple pregnancy and tumours of the genital tract. The size of the fetus is appropriate for gestation. For each item listed below, choose the **single**

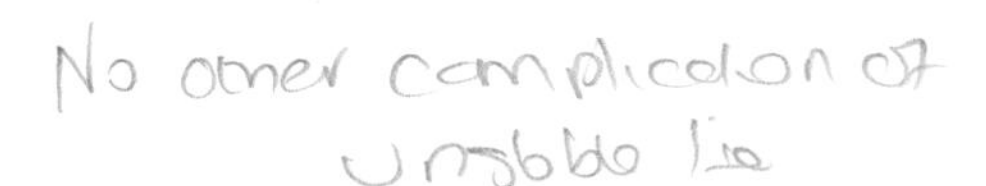

most appropriate option for management. Each option may be used once, more than once or not at all.

Item 1 ▶ The pregnant woman is 40 years old, 40 weeks pregnant and is contracting 1 in 3 with intact membranes and transverse lie of the fetus.
Answer ▷ *H*=Lower-segment caesarean section.

Item 2 ▶ The pregnant woman is at a gestation of 40 weeks and 10 days; she is not contracting, the membranes are intact and the lie of the fetus is oblique, with the head in the left iliac fossa.
Answer ▷ *I*=Stabilising induction of labour.

Item 3 ▶ The pregnant woman has reached a gestation of 40 weeks and 10 days; she is not contracting, the membranes are intact and the lie of the fetus is transverse. One of the previous deliveries was by lower-segment caesarean section for breech presentation.
Answer ▷ *H*=Lower-segment caesarean section.

Item 4 ▶ The woman is 32 years old, at a gestation of 39 weeks and was admitted 2 days ago for unstable lie. However, the fetus had been in longitudinal lie since admission and presenting by the head with intact membranes.
Answer ▷ *A*=Allow home.

Item 5 ▶ The woman is 34 years old, at a gestation of 38 weeks, the fetal lie is unstable, the membranes are intact and there are no contractions. Her first delivery was by uncomplicated lower-segment caesarean section for breech presentation.
Answer ▷ *C*=Await spontaneous labour following admission.

Item 6 ▶ The woman is 34 years old, the pregnancy has reached a gestation of 39 weeks, the fetal lie is unstable, the membranes are intact and there are no uterine contractions. There was a history of moderate self-limiting antepartum

haemorrhage at 32 weeks during this pregnancy.
Answer ▷ *H* = Lower-segment caesarean section.

Commentary

Purpose

In this EMQ, the examiners wish to test your understanding of the management of unstable lie during pregnancy.

Content

There are ten options followed by a lead-in statement. The lead-in statement acts as the bridge between the list of ten options and the six items. The pregnant woman is described very clearly as being: healthy, with three living children, all of whom were delivered normally (unless otherwise stated); she is pregnant for the fourth time; the lie of the fetus is unstable and there is no evidence of placenta praevia, polyhydramnios, uterine malformation, fetal abnormality, multiple pregnancy or tumours of the genital tract. It is stated clearly that the size of the baby is appropriate for gestation. Because of the way the question is focused, there is no room for ambiguity. Your correct answers to this question would demonstrate:

1. Your understanding of the management of women with unstable lie of the fetus.
2. Your safety as a clinician.

Answers

Item 1 = *H* ▶ A pregnant woman who is in labour at term with intact membranes and transverse lie of the fetus must be delivered forthwith by lower segment caesarean section; therefore, the answer to *Item 1* is *H*.

Item 2 = *I* ▶ In this question, the pregnant woman is at a gestation of 40 weeks and 10 days. Therefore, delivery would need to be considered on the grounds of post-dates pregnancy. The pregnant woman is not in labour, the membranes are intact and the lie of the fetus is oblique, with the head in the left iliac fossa. Under these circumstances, the most appropriate management would be to attempt stabilising induction of labour. Therefore, the answer is *I*.

Item 3 = H ▶ In this scenario, the pregnant woman has reached a point in gestation – 40 weeks and 10 days – where delivery would need to be considered; she is not in labour, the lie of the fetus is transverse and the examiners point you further in the right direction by mentioning that one of the previous deliveries was by lower-segment caesarean section for breech presentation. Therefore, the answer is *H*, delivery by lower-segment caesarean section.

Item 4 = A ▶ If the lie of the baby has stabilised spontaneously and the lie of the fetus has been longitudinal for 2 days, the most appropriate management would be to allow the woman to go home. Therefore, the answer is *A*.

Item 5 = C ▶ In this scenario, the woman is 34 years old, her pregnancy has reached a gestation of 38 weeks with unstable lie of the fetus and the woman is not in labour. Her first delivery was by lower-segment caesarean section for breech presentation. The examiners helpfully state that the caesarean section was uncomplicated. A trial of labour for vaginal birth following a previous caesarean section would be a reasonable option. There is no indication to expedite delivery at 38 weeks and spontaneous onset of labour may well result in spontaneous version to longitudinal lie and vertex presentation.

Item 6 = H ▶ The history of moderate self-limiting antepartum haemorrhage at 32 weeks of gestation has the following implications:

1. The pregnancy is best ended by delivery of a healthy infant no later than a gestational age of 39 weeks.
2. Manipulative actions such as stabilising induction

are best avoided with a history of antepartum haemorrhage. Therefore, the answer is *H*.

Minimising risk and maximising your score

This is a relatively straightforward question and the examiners have pointed the candidates in the right direction by providing a lot of information. The gestation in each scenario is presented and the obstetric histories are clearly written. The list of options does contain some functional distractors but these can be easily dismissed. Candidates who take into account all of the information that is provided in each question would have little difficulty in arriving at the correct answer.

Controversy may arise over *Item 5*. Why is the answer not *H*? There is no reason to expedite delivery at 38 weeks. The lead-in statement explains that there are no underlying causes for the unstable lie. If the woman's age was a risk factor or the pregnancy was more advanced than 38 weeks then *H* would be the answer.

STEM/OPTION LIST 8

Theme ▷ Obstetrics: prenatal diagnosis of Down syndrome.

Domain ▷ Diagnosis, investigations.

Options

- A Amniocentesis at 13 weeks
- B Amniocentesis at 16 weeks for karyotype
- C Amniocentesis for level of insulin in amniotic fluid
- D Amniocentesis for the detection of level of AFP
- E Chorionic villus biopsy at 11 weeks for karyotype
- F Cordocentesis at 19 weeks for karyotype
- G Fetoscopy and fetal liver biopsy at 19 weeks
- H Fetoscopy and fetal skin biopsy at 19 weeks

I No further action
J Placental biopsy at 20 weeks for karyotype and immunohistochemistry

Instructions

Each of the clinical situations described below concerns a pregnant woman who wishes to consider prenatal diagnosis of Down syndrome, having undergone the appropriate counselling. There is no family history of Down syndrome. For each item, choose the **single** most appropriate option for management. Each option may be used once, more than once or not at all.

Item 1 ▶ The woman is a 24-year-old primigravida at 16 weeks of gestation. Antenatal screening for Down syndrome by serological tests and measurement of nuchal thickness shows a risk of 1 in 5000.
Answer ▷ *I*=No further action.

Item 2 ▶ The woman is a 21-year-old primigravida at 16 weeks of gestation and serum screening for Down syndrome has shown a risk of 1 in 120.
Answer ▷ *B*=Amniocentesis at 16 weeks for karyotype.

Item 3 ▶ The woman is 46 years old, is pregnant for the fourth time, has three healthy children and is 10 weeks of gestation.
Answer ▷ *E*=Chorionic villus biopsy at 11 weeks for karyotype.

Item 4 ▶ The woman is 40 years old, she has one healthy child, this is her second pregnancy and the pregnancy has reached 16 weeks. The results of antenatal serum screening for Down syndrome (without nuchal thickness measurement) show a risk of 1 in 300. It is brought to your attention that this woman's serum sample was sent by mistake to the serology laboratory with the woman's age listed as 20 years old.
Answer ▷ *B*=Amniocentesis at 16 weeks for karyotype.

Item 5 ▶ The woman is a 42-year-old primigravida at a gestation of 13 weeks.
Answer ▷ *B* = Amniocentesis at 16 weeks for karyotype.

Item 6 ▶ The woman is aged 28 years, this is her second pregnancy, which has reached a gestational age of 10 weeks; she has previously undergone termination of pregnancy for Down syndrome. Genetic testing has shown that she has a balanced translocation 14:21 and her partner has a normal karyotype.
Answer ▷ *E* = Chorionic villus biopsy at 11 weeks for karyotype.

Commentary

Purpose

To probe your understanding of the systems for prenatal diagnosis of Down syndrome.

Content

This EMQ has ten options – a lead-in statement and six items. Several of the options are obvious distractors – measurement of level of insulin in amniotic fluid, fetal skin biopsy and fetal liver biopsy. Once you have read the lead-in statement and considered each item it should be easy to answer the items without looking through the whole list of options. Time is saved by avoiding distractors.

Answers

Item 1 = I ▶ This 24-year-old primigravida is at low risk, therefore, the answer is *I*.

Item 2 = B ▶ This 21-year-old primigravida is 'screen positive' and therefore, the option is *B*.

Item 3 = E ▶ This 46-year-old woman has an age related risk which would warrant the consideration of chorionic villous biopsy at 11 weeks. Therefore, the answer is *E*.

Item 4 = *B* ▶ This 40-year-old woman has an age-related risk of Down syndrome which is significant. This particular item contains a distractor that is based on erroneous serum screening – the woman's age is incorrectly entered – therefore, the answer is *B*.

Item 5 = *B* ▶ This 42-year-old primigravida has a significant age-related risk of having a child with Down syndrome. The gestational age is 13 weeks, which is generally considered to be rather late for chorionic villus sampling. Therefore, the answer is *B*.

Item 6 = *E* ▶ This young woman with a balanced translocation 14 : 21, with a partner who has a normal karyotype, has a significant chance of having a child with Down syndrome. If the 14 : 21 balanced translocation is found in the woman, the risk of a chromosomally unbalanced child is 15%. Therefore, the answer is *E*.

Minimising risk and maximising your score

This is a very straightforward question and it is important not to misread the numbers. Pay particular attention to the woman's age in each item, the gestational age of her pregnancy and (where provided) the level of risk. It is also important to note whether or not the level of risk has been measured correctly. For example, *Item 4* describes a woman whose age has been entered into the request form incorrectly. This EMQ also illustrates the fact that the answers must be taken from the list of options. You may well have another form of valid management in your own mind. However, the answers to most of the items are obvious and you would be able to judge exactly what to do and then choose the appropriate option from the list of options.

STEM/OPTION LIST 9

Theme ▷ Gynaecology, perimenopausal contraception.

Domain ▷ Management.

Options

A Advise combined hormone replacement therapy
B Advise endometrial sampling prior to decision
C Arrange a progesterone withdrawal test prior to decision
D Check mid-luteal serum progesterone before decision
E Check preovulatory serum LH surge before decision
F Check serum FSH during menstruation before decision
G Check serum LH before decision
H Continue using contraception for a further 3 months
I Continue using contraception for a further 6 months
J Continue using contraception for a further 6 months and then stop if the total duration of amenorrhoea since the last spontaneous menses is 1 year
K Continue using contraception for a further 2 years and then stop if the total duration of amenorrhoea since the last spontaneous menses is 3 years
L Continue using contraception for a further 5 years
M Continue using contraception until anovulation is confirmed by endocrine tests
N Measure serum prolactin and serum FSH before decision
O Stop using contraception
P Stop using contraception if BMI is less than 22

Instructions

The scenarios described below refer to a healthy woman who wishes to ascertain whether or not she should stop using contraception. Select the **single** most appropriate piece of advice for each woman from the list of options. Each option may be used once, more than once or not at all.

Item 1 ▶ The woman is aged 55 years and her last spontaneous menstrual period was 2 years ago.
Answer ▷ O = Stop using contraception.

Item 2 ▶ The woman is aged 53 years and her last spontaneous menstrual period was 25 months ago.
Answer ▷ O = Stop using contraception.

Item 3 ▶ The woman is aged 51 years and her last spontaneous menstrual period was 6 months ago.
Answer ▷ *J* = Continue using contraception for a further 6 months and then stop if the total duration of amenorrhoea since the last spontaneous menses is 1 year.

Commentary

Purpose

This EMQ is designed to test a candidate's understanding of when to stop contraception in a perimenopausal woman.

Content

There are 16 options followed by a lead-in statement, which explains clearly that the scenarios refer to a healthy woman who wishes to ascertain whether or not she should stop using contraception. There are three items that describe different women and you are asked to select the most appropriate piece of advice from the list of options.

The key points to understand are as follows:

1. A woman may be advised to stop using contraception 2 years after her last spontaneous menstrual period if she is aged under 50 years.
2. A woman may be advised to stop using contraception 1 year after her last spontaneous menstrual period if she is aged 50 years or over.

Therefore, the answer in each case to *Items 1* and *2* is *O*. The answer to *Item 3* is *J*.

Minimising risk and maximising your score

This is an example of a question with multiple distractors for each correct item/option match. Many of the alternate options would simply not be considered in the day to day running of a clinic. However, is option *I* an answer to *Item 3*? Option *I* would be an incorrect choice, as the 51-year-old woman referred to in *Item 3* may menstruate spontaneously shortly after she consults you for advice. Option *A* refers to hormone replacement therapy, which is not contraceptive in function. Reading the lead-in statement properly dismisses it as a distractor.

STEM/OPTION LIST 10

Theme ▷ Gynaecology: contraception, progestogen-based.

Domain ▷ Pharmacology, prescribing administration, management.

Options

A Twice daily
B Once daily
C Once daily between day 14 and day 28 of each menstrual cycle
D Once daily between day 5 and day 24 of each menstrual cycle
E Once daily for 21 days followed by a 7-day break
F Once on alternate days
G Twice weekly
H Once weekly
I Once every 4 weeks
J Twice every 12 weeks
K Once every 8 weeks
L Once every 12 weeks
M Once every 16 weeks
N Once immediately
O Once followed by a second dose 48 hours later
P Once followed by a second dose 72 hours later

Instructions

The following items refer to progestogen-only contraception, which is to be used in women who have no contraindications to their use and who have chosen the method following appropriate counselling. For each item listed below, choose the **single** most appropriate frequency of administration from the list of options above. Each option may be used once, more than once or not at all.

Item 1 ▶ Desogestrel.
Answer ▷ *B* = Once daily.

Item 2 ▶ Etynodiol.
Answer ▷ *B* = Once daily.

Item 3 ▶ Norethisterone enantate (oily).
Answer ▷ *K* = Once every 8 weeks.

Item 4 ▶ Medroxyprogesterone acetate aqueous suspension.
Answer ▷ *L* = Once every 12 weeks.

Item 5 ▶ Medroxyprogesterone acetate aqueous suspension for a woman taking carbamazepine.
Answer ▷ *L* = Once every 12 weeks.

Commentary

Purpose

This EMQ tests a candidate's understanding of the use of progestogen-only contraception.

Content

There are 16 options followed by a lead-in statement that makes it absolutely clear that the subsequent items refer to progestogen-only contraception. Furthermore the lead-in statement makes it quite clear that the progestogen-only contraception is to be used in women with no contraindications to their use. It is also made clear that the women have chosen the method following appropriate counselling and the candidate is simply asked to choose the most appropriate frequency of administration from the list of options.

Answers

Desogestrel and etynodiol refer to different formulations of progestogen-only pills. Therefore, the answers to *Items 1* and *2* is *B*.

Item 3 = *K*.
Item 4 = *L*.

The concurrent use of pharmacological agents that induce liver enzymes does not appear to affect the efficacy of medroxyprogesterone acetate aqueous suspension. Therefore, the frequency of administration of medroxyprogesterone acetate aqueous suspension need not be altered for women taking carbamazepine. Hence, the answer to *Item 5* is also *L*.

Minimising risk and maximising your score

It is important to be familiar with the pharmacological names of the drugs that you commonly prescribe. It is also important to be aware of different drug interactions and whether or not the frequency of administration needs to be altered with the concurrent use of certain other drugs. Overall, this is a very straightforward question and illustrates how the lead-in statement removes any ambiguity in explaining to the candidate what is required.

STEM/OPTION LIST 11

Theme ▷ Management of infertility.

Domain ▷ Audit.

Options

A Application of Caldicott principles
B Benchmarking
C Change management
D Incorporation of consistency checks

E Measure of outcome
F Measure of process
G Measure of structure
H Re-audit
I Review criterion
J Standard and target level of performance

Instructions

Your department decides to conduct an audit of the management of women with infertility. The following items refer to various steps in the audit cycle. For each item described below, select the **single** most appropriate match from the list of options above. Each option may be used once, more than once or not at all.

Item 1 ▶ It is stated that all women with anovulatory cycles must undergo measurement of serum prolactin.
Answer ▷ *I* = Review criterion.

Item 2 ▶ The investigators and data collectors ensure that patient-identifiable information is handled properly and responsibly.
Answer ▷ *A* = Application of Caldicott principles.

Item 3 ▶ Analysis of data from the pilot study shows a mean age of 54 years and that women with primary infertility had a history of previous caesarean section. The investigators require a method for crosschecking their data entry.
Answer ▷ *D* = Incorporation of consistency checks.

Item 4 ▶ Once the findings are presented, it is agreed that the appropriate referral of women to the Regional Centre for Assisted Reproduction within 6 months of first attendance in clinic is an attainable goal.
Answer ▷ *B* = Benchmarking.

Commentary

Purpose

The purpose of this EMQ is to test the candidate's understanding of the terminology of clinical audit.

Content

There are TEN options, which correspond with various stages of the audit cycle, but they are not necessarily in order. The lead-in statement describes how the candidate's department decides to conduct an audit of the management of women with infertility. There are four items and the candidate is asked to select the most appropriate match for each statement from the list of options.

Answers

Item 1 = I ▶ Review criterion. This is a specific healthcare statement, which can be subject to audit.

Item 2 = A ▶ The Caldicott principles consist of several points which data collectors and investigators must follow in order to preserve the confidentiality of patients.

Item 3 = D ▶ It is clear that the data are contradictory, therefore consistency checks must be incorporated.

Item 4 = B ▶ Benchmarking is the process of defining an attainable goal. In this case, the findings are presented and it is agreed that the appropriate referral of women to the Regional Centre for Assisted Reproduction within 6 months of first attendance in clinic is an attainable goal. Benchmarking is more generalised than a review criterion.

Minimising risk and maximising your score

It is essential that you understand the audit cycle and basic terminology that is used in clinical audit. Most of the distractors in the list of options can be dismissed easily. A candidate may disagree with a certain proposal for management or a certain timeframe for valid reasons but these are irrelevant to answering the EMQ.

STEM/OPTION LIST 12

Theme ▷ Gynaecology: surgery.

Domain ▷ Clinical prioritisation, management.

Options

A Arrange chest X-ray, if results are normal then proceed
B Cancel the operation
C Defer operation and discuss at a multidisciplinary case conference
D Defer for 1 week
E Defer for 2 weeks
F Defer for 1 month
G Defer for 6 months
H Discharge woman, treat infection, readmit
I Discuss with anaesthetist
J Proceed on an emergency basis
K Proceed with the operation as planned
L Treat infection and defer the operation for 2 days

Instructions

Each of the following clinical scenarios refers to a woman who is scheduled to undergo surgery for various reasons. However, you are asked to review the timing of the operation in the light of clinical circumstances described. Choose the **single** most appropriate management from the list of options for each of the items listed below. Each option may be used once, more than once or not at all.

Item 1 ▶ A 30-year-old woman has been admitted for day case laparoscopic sterilisation. You are informed that the

woman has been vomiting and there is a pelvic mass.
Answer ▷ *B*=Cancel the operation.

Item 2 ▶ A 26-year-old woman returned from a long vacation in South India and has been admitted for daycase laparoscopy and dye test. The woman has been feeling unwell for several days with headache, malaise and intermittent fever.
Answer ▷ *B*=Cancel the operation.

Item 3 ▶ A 23-year-old woman has been admitted to the ward with unequivocal features of a ruptured tubal pregnancy; her blood pressure is 75/45 mmHg with a pulse rate of 112 beats/minute and the peripheries are cold. One week previously the woman had attended her general practitioner's surgery as she had symptoms of a sore throat. The woman was treated for a streptococcal infection of the pharynx but methicillin-resistant *Staphylococcus aureus* (MSRA) was isolated from a nasal swab taken in the surgery a week ago.
Answer ▷ *J*=Proceed on an emergency basis.

Item 4 ▶ A 35-year-old woman has been admitted to undergo radical hysterectomy for invasive cancer of the cervix. A profuse growth of beta-haemolytic streptococcus of Lancefield group B was isolated by culture from a high vaginal swab taken from the woman 1 week previously.
Answer ▷ *K*=Proceed with the operation as planned.

Item 5 ▶ A 30-year-old woman has been admitted to undergo daycase diagnostic laparoscopy for the investigation of pelvic pain and is noted to have cellulitis and a small abscess at the site of an umbilical ring. The umbilical ring had been removed by the woman herself 2 weeks previously, after she was seen in clinic by a very helpful junior doctor who had answered some questions the woman wanted to ask prior to the operation. MSRA has been isolated by culture from a swab taken 2 weeks ago from the small abscess and the report is shown to you after admission.
Answer ▷ *H*=Discharge woman, treat infection, readmit.

Commentary

Purpose

This EMQ is designed to test a candidate's ability to prioritise clinical issues in gynaecology and to make decisions.

Content

There are 12 options, a lead-in statement, which explains clearly that the candidate is asked to review the timing of the operation, and five different items, with each one referring to a different clinical scenario.

Answers

Item 1 = B ▶ A 30-year-old woman is being admitted for what is obviously a non-urgent laparoscopic sterilisation. The woman may well be pregnant as she has been vomiting and she has a pelvic mass. There would certainly be this suspicion at the very least. Therefore, the answer is *B*.

Item 2 = B ▶ This 26-year-old woman, who has returned from a long vacation in South India, is being admitted for a non-urgent operation. The woman, who has developed a feeling of being unwell with headache, malaise and intermittent fever, may well have malaria. Therefore, the answer is *B*.

Item 3 = J ▶ This 23-year-old woman has nasal carriage of MRSA. However, she also has a life-threatening gynaecological emergency. Therefore, the answer is *J*.

Item 4 = K ▶ This 35-year-old woman is about to undergo radical surgery for invasive cancer of the cervix. The presence of group B streptococcus in the vagina may indicate colonisation and it may well be very difficult to eradicate the organism from the vagina in the presence of an invasive cancer of the cervix. Almost certainly, this woman would be receiving perioperative antibiotics and therefore, the answer is *K*.

Item 5 = H ▶ This 30-year-old woman has MRSA, which was isolated from an abscess in the region of the umbilicus. The woman was scheduled to undergo a non-urgent operation and therefore the priority would be to defer the operation until the abscess has been treated and resolved. Therefore, the answer is *H*.

Minimising risk and maximising your score

This is an example of an EMQ where clinical experience rather than 'book knowledge' is required. It is also important to note that the candidate is asked to review the timing of the operation in the light of clinical circumstances and then choose the most appropriate management from the list of options. This question is **not** a test of a candidate's diagnostic ability as such. Consider, for example, *Items 1* and *2*. A 30-year-old woman with vomiting and a pelvic mass generates an extremely long differential diagnosis. The EMQ does not ask the candidate to consider the various diagnostic possibilities. The candidate is asked to make a decision on the timing of the operation in the light of clinical circumstances. A non-urgent operation such as laparoscopic sterilisation must be cancelled. In *Item 2*, a 26-year-old woman returning from a long vacation in South India may well have malaria but again the differential diagnosis is long. It is unlikely that the laparoscopy and dye test would be useful in determining the diagnosis. The non-urgent operation must be cancelled and not merely deferred within a certain timeframe. A candidate may well wonder why option *H* may not be an answer. Although malaria is an infection, there is no evidence from the information given that the woman does indeed have malaria. Therefore, the single best answer is best represented in option *B*. Candidates who attempt this EMQ should remain focused on exactly what has been asked in the EMQ and avoid the distractors.

STEM/OPTION LIST 13

Theme ▷ Gynaecology: oncology.

Domain ▷ Diagnosis.

Options

	Age (years)	Chief symptom(s)	Salient clinical and radiological findings	Clinical chemistry
A	18	Pelvic pain	Pelvic mass	Elevated serum αFP Elevated serum alpha-1 antitrypsin
B	18	Irregular vaginal bleeding Pelvic pain Blindness No history of recent pregnancy	Pelvic mass Intracranial space-occupying lesion	Elevated serum βhCG Normal serum αFP and CA125
C	14	Vaginal bleeding Precocious puberty	Pelvic mass	Elevated serum βhCG Elevated serum αFP
D	40	Postcoital bleeding	Necrotic mass in upper vagina Tumour-free space between lesion and pelvic sidewall No hydronephrosis	Normal serum αFP, βhCG, CA125

	Age (years)	Chief symptom(s)	Salient clinical and radiological findings	Clinical chemistry
E	50	Postcoital bleeding	Necrotic mass in upper vagina No tumour-free space between lesion and pelvic sidewall Unilateral hydronephrosis	Normal serum αFP, βhCG, CA125
F	60	Abdominal distension	Pelvic mass, ascites, stellate masses in omentum	Elevated serum CA125
G	40	Postcoital bleeding Sallow appearance	Pelvic mass with infiltration into the rectum Rectal ulceration Bilateral hydronephrosis	Normal serum CA125, αFP, βhCG
H	60		Bulky uterus with increased endometrial thickening	Normal serum CA125, αFP, HLG
I	52		Bulky uterus, increased endometrial thickening Unilateral adnexal mass with a diameter of 12 cm	Elevated serum inhibin. Serum FSH in the premenopausal range Normal serum CA125, αFP, βhCG
J	25	Irregular vaginal bleeding Early virilisation	Solid adnexal mass with a diameter of 6 cm	Elevated serum testosterone, normal serum CA125, αFP, βhCG

Instructions

For each of the following gynaecological malignancies, select the **single** most appropriate tumour profile from the list of options in the table above. Each option may be used once, more than once or not at all.

Item 1 ▶ Endodermal sinus tumour.
Answer ▷ *A* = (18 years/Pelvic pain/Pelvic mass/Elevated serum α-fetoprotein, elevated serum α-1 antitrypsin).

Item 2 ▶ Nongestational choriocarcinoma of the ovary.
Answer ▷ *B* = (18 years/Irregular vaginal bleeding, pelvic pain, blindness, no history of recent pregnancy/Pelvic mass, Intracranial space-occupying lesion/Elevated serum βhCG, normal serum αFP and CA125.

Item 3 ▶ Embryonal carcinoma of the ovary.
Answer ▷ *C* = (14 years/Vaginal bleeding, precocious puberty/Pelvic mass/Elevated serum βhCG, elevated serum αFP.

Commentary

Purpose

This EMQ is designed to probe your understanding of diagnostic oncology. Do you understand the chief clinical, radiological and biochemical features of various gynaecological malignancies?

Content

The EMQ consists of ten options, each of which represents a different tumour profile. The lead-in statement is suitably short and merely asks you to match the different gynaecological malignancies listed in the items with the appropriate option.

Answers

Item 1 = A ▶ Endodermal sinus tumour affects relatively young women who have pelvic pain, a pelvic mass and an elevated serum αFP. The serum α-1 antitrypsin level is often elevated in these patients and therefore, the answer is *A*. Even if you are unable to recall the exact clinical features of this relatively rare tumour, most candidates would know that endodermal sinus tumour is associated with an elevated serum αFP. If you do need to read all the options then you would realise that there are only two options (*A* and *C*) where the serum αFP is elevated. Endodermal sinus tumour is not associated with either precocious puberty or an elevated serum βhCG. Therefore, the answer must be *A*.

Item 2 = B ▶ Non-gestational ovarian choriocarcinoma is exceedingly rare and the answer is *B*. This particular malignancy is not associated with a recent history of pregnancy; it affects younger women; early metastases occur and the serum αhCG is significantly elevated.

Item 3 = C ▶ Embryonal carcinoma of the ovary is rare and it is a cause of precocious puberty. The serum βhCG and serum αFP are both elevated. The answer is *C*.

Minimising risk and maximising your score

There is no need to feel intimidated by the presence in the examination of rare conditions. Although it is recommended that the 'best' technique for passing the EMQs is to read the lead-in statement, consider each item, have a mental picture of the likely answer and then select the answer from the list of options, this is an example of an EMQ where it may be useful to read through the options. The number of distractors for each item/option match is actually quite low.

STEM/OPTION LIST 14

Theme ▷ Research methodology: antenatal screening.

Domain ▷ Statistics.

Options

A	125.00	H	79.00
B	100.00	I	77.00
C	90.40	J	16.88
D	90.00	K	15.46
E	83.00	L	13.39
F	81.00	M	5.00
G	80.00	N	2.50

In a prospective blind study of a possible new method of antenatal fetal screening for a particular disorder, 5000 pregnant women rated as having a high risk for babies with this disorder were recruited and tested. These were the results:

	Baby born with disorder	**Baby born without disorder**	**Totals**
Tested positive	200	475	675
Tested negative	50	4275	4325
Totals	**250**	**4750**	**5000**

Instructions

For each situation described below, choose the **single** most appropriate figure (rounded to two decimal points) from the above list. Each option may be used once, more than once, or not at all.

Item 1 ▶ The percentage chance of a woman with a positive screening test having a child affected by the disorder.
Answer ▷ G=80.00.

Item 2 ▶ The positive predictive value.
Answer ▷ G = 80.00.

Commentary

Purpose

Medical statistics almost always make a brief appearance in MRCOG papers to check candidates' understanding of them. This EMQ tests candidates' knowledge of statistical definitions and their ability to perform simple statistical calculations.

Answers

Item 1 = G ▶ The percentage chance of a woman with a positive test having a child affected by the disorder screened for requires a simple rate calculation. This is completed by dividing the total tested positive and born with the disorder (200) by the total born with the disorder (200 ÷ 250 = 0.8, 0.8 × 100% = 80%).

Item 1 = G ▶ *Item 1* describes the 'positive predictive value', so again *Item 2* is the total tested positive and born with disorder (200) divided by the total born with the disorder (200 ÷ 250 = 0.8, 0.8 × 100% = 80%).

Minimising risk and maximising your score

These are relatively easy calculations but they need to be 'got right'. There are distractors, so checking your maths is recommended. As in previous questions, there is quite a lot of information that is totally superfluous in the table, so cutting to the chase and quickly honing in on only that information required to complete the task and the answer will save useful time.

STEM/OPTION LIST 15

Theme ▷ Research methodology: antenatal screening.

Domain ▷ Statistics.

Options

A	125.00	H	66.67
B	100.00	I	25.00
C	90.40	J	22.50
D	90.00	K	11.11
E	88.00	L	10.00
F	85.00	M	6.25
G	80.00	N	4.76

In a prospective blind study of a possible new method of antenatal fetal screening for a particular disorder, 2100 pregnant women rated as having a high risk for babies with this disorder were recruited and tested. These were the results:

	Baby born with disorder	**Baby born without disorder**	**Totals**
Tested positive	90	400	490
Tested negative	10	1600	1610
Totals	**100**	**2000**	**2100**

Instructions

For each situation described below, choose the **single** most appropriate figure (rounded to two decimal points) from the above list. Each option may be used once, more than once, or not at all.

Item 1 ▶ The specificity of the test.
Answer ▷ *G*=80.00%.

Item 2 ▶ The sensitivity of the test.
Answer ▷ *D*=90.00%.

Commentary

Purpose

Like the last one, this EMQ tests candidates' knowledge of statistical definitions and their ability to perform statistical calculations. The calculations are little more complex but the definitions are again central to medical statistics, and all candidates should know them. The main purpose of the test it to know that you precisely and actively know what specificity and sensitivity mean.

Answers

Item 1 = G ▶ The specificity is the proportion of normals which the test calls normal – the proportion of true negatives (1600 ÷ 2000 = 80.00%).

Item 2 = D ▶ Sensitivity is the number of true positives divided by the true positives plus the false negatives (90 ÷ [90 + 10] = 90 ÷ 100 = 90.00%).

Minimising risk and maximising your score

This question represents about the maximum degree of difficulty of calculation expected of candidates in the examination. After all, calculators are not allowed. The distractors allow for the catching out of candidates doing the wrong calculations – in a number of different ways. An important tip to take from this is that getting to an answer that is on the list of options does not mean that it is right. If writing out the maths will make you do it more accurately, do so.

4 | Mock examination 1

STEM/OPTION LIST 1

Options

A Bladder irrigation
B Bolus subcutaneous injection; repeated
C Bolus subcutaneous injection; immediately
D Continuous intravenous infusion
E Continuous subcutaneous infusion
F Implant
G Inhalation of a nebulised spray
H Intramuscular
I Intrathecal
J Intravenous injection
K Nasal drops
L Per oram
M Per vaginam
N Retention enema
O Sublingual
P Topical application
Q Via central venous line
R Via nasogastric tube

Instructions

The following scenarios refer to women who require treatment or palliation for various conditions. Select the **single** most appropriate route of administration for the pharmacological agent which is to be used from the list of options. Each option may be used once, more than once or not at all.

Questions

1 ▷ A woman is undergoing cytotoxic chemotherapy for ovarian cancer in the appropriate centre. As part of the regimen, cisplatin needs to be given.

2 ▷ A pregnant woman has eclampsia and magnesium needs to be given.

3 ▷ A pregnant woman is about to undergo elective caesarean section and magnesium trisilicate mixture needs to be given.

4 ▷ A pregnant woman has undergone appendicectomy under general anaesthesia, following which there are signs of opiate-induced respiratory depression and naloxone must be given.

STEM/OPTION LIST 2

Options

A Acute maternal CMV with equivocal evidence of fetal infection
B Acute maternal toxocara infection
C Acute maternal toxoplasmosis
D Acute maternal toxoplasmosis infection with equivocal evidence of fetal infection
E Acute maternal toxoplasmosis infection with fetal infection
F Acute maternal toxoplasmosis infection with no fetal infection
G Acute maternal tularaemia
H Chronic maternal CMV infection
I Chronic maternal toxocara infection
J Maternal Q fever
K No evidence of maternal toxoplasmosis
L Previous maternal toxoplasmosis

Instructions

The following clinical scenarios refer to a pregnant woman who has previously been in good health and who has developed headache, fever, fatigue and sore throat. The outstanding clinical sign on examination is generalised lymphadenopathy. The results of various investigations are provided in the items below. For each item, choose the **single** most likely diagnosis from the list of options. Each option may be used once, more than once or not at all.

Questions

5 ▷ Sabin-Feldman dye test is positive at high titre and the corresponding IgM titre is positive at high titre in maternal serum.

6 ▷ Sabin-Feldman dye test is positive at low titre and the corresponding IgM, IgE and IgA are undetected in maternal serum. Three weeks later the tests are repeated and the Sabin-Feldman test is positive, the IgM is positive at high titre and the corresponding IgE and IgA are detectable.

STEM/OPTION LIST 3

Options

A	0	I	1 in 8
B	1 in 250	J	1 in 4
C	1 in 100	K	2 in 7
D	1 in 28	L	1 in 3
E	1 in 25	M	3 in 8
F	1 in 20	N	3 in 7
G	1 in 16	O	1 in 2
H	1 in 12	P	2 in 3

Instructions

A pregnant woman consults you for advice, as there is a family history of congenital adrenal hyperplasia. Genetic and biochemical studies show that the woman and her partner are carriers of 21-hydroxylsase deficiency. The woman has a question, which is listed in the item below. Select the **single** most appropriate answer to the question from the above list of options.

Question

7 ▷ What is the risk of an affected daughter in this pregnancy?

STEM/OPTION LIST 4

Options

A	0	I	1 in 3
B	1 in 100	J	4 in 10
C	1 in 88	K	1 in 2
D	1 in 25	L	2 in 3
E	1 in 16	M	3 to 1
F	1 in 8	N	2 to 1
G	1 in 4	O	3 to 2
H	3 in 10	P	1 in 1

Instructions

A man with vitamin D-resistant rickets has three affected children. Unfortunately, his first wife, with whom he had these children, died a few years ago. He has since remarried. His new wife is a healthy woman, who is now pregnant with the man's baby, and she consults you. The woman asks you various questions concerning the risks to her baby. The item refers to one of the woman's questions. Select the **single** most appropriate answer to the woman's question from the list of options above.

Question

8 ▷ If the baby is affected in this pregnancy, what is the risk of having an affected child in the next pregnancy?

STEM/OPTION LIST 5

Options

- A Amniocentesis at 13 weeks
- B Amniocentesis at 16 weeks for karyotype
- C Amniocentesis for level of insulin in amniotic fluid
- D Amniocentesis for the detection of level of αFP
- E Chorionic villus biopsy at 11 weeks for karyotype
- F Cordocentesis at 19 weeks for karyotype
- G Fetoscopy and fetal liver biopsy at 19 weeks
- H Fetoscopy and fetal skin biopsy at 19 weeks
- I No further action
- J Placental biopsy at 20 weeks for karyotype and immunohistochemistry

Instructions

Each of the clinical situations described below concerns a pregnant woman who wishes to undergo prenatal diagnosis of Down syndrome, having undergone the appropriate counselling. For each item, choose the **single** most appropriate option for management. Each option may be used once, more than once or not at all.

Questions

9 ▷ The woman is a 38-year-old primigravida at a gestation of 13 weeks, who has insulin-dependent diabetes mellitus.

10 ▷ The woman is a 24-year-old primigravida at a gestation of 16 weeks. She has a niece with Down syndrome. Genetic tests have demonstrated that the niece's parents have a normal karyotype. The woman has undergone nuchal thickness measurement and serum screening for Down syndrome, which show a risk of 1 in 500.

STEM/OPTION LIST 6

Options

A Advise combined hormone replacement therapy
B Advise endometrial sampling prior to decision
C Arrange a progesterone withdrawal test prior to decision
D Check mid-luteal serum progesterone before decision
E Check preovulatory serum LH surge before decision
F Check serum FSH during menstruation before decision
G Check serum LH before decision
H Continue using contraception for a further 3 months
I Continue using contraception for a further 6 months
J Continue using contraception for a further 6 months and then stop if the total duration of amenorrhoea since the last spontaneous menses is 1 year
K Continue using contraception for a further 2 years and then stop if the total duration of amenorrhoea since the last spontaneous menses is 3 years
L Continue using contraception for a further 5 years
M Continue using contraception until anovulation is confirmed by endocrine tests
N Measure serum prolactin and serum FSH before decision
O Stop using contraception
P Stop using contraception if BMI is less than 22

Instructions

The scenarios described below refer to a healthy woman who wishes to ascertain whether or not she should stop using contraception. Select the **single** most appropriate piece of advice for each woman from the list of options a below. Each option may be used once, more than once or not at all.

Questions

11 ▷ The woman is aged 48 years and her last spontaneous menstrual period was 3 years ago.

12 ▷ The woman is aged 52 years and her last spontaneous menstrual period was 18 months ago.

STEM/OPTION LIST 7

Options

A Twice daily
B Once daily
C Once daily between day 14 and day 28 of each menstrual cycle
D Once daily between day 5 and day 24 of each menstrual cycle
E Once daily for 21 days followed by a 7-day break
F Once on alternate days
G Twice weekly
H Once weekly
I Once every 4 weeks
J Twice every 12 weeks
K Once every 8 weeks
L Once every 12 weeks
M Once every 16 weeks
N Once stat
O Once followed by a second dose 48 hours later
P Once followed by a second dose 72 hours later

Instructions

The following items refer to progestogen-only contraception, which is to be used in women who have no contraindications to their use and who have chosen the method following appropriate counselling. For each item listed below choose the **single** most appropriate frequency of administration from the list of options above. Each option may be used once, more than once or not at all.

Questions

13 ▷ Norethisterone.

14 ▷ Medroxyprogesterone acetate aqueous suspension for a woman taking rifampicin.

15 ▷ Medroxyprogesterone acetate aqueous suspension for a woman taking griseofulvin.

STEM/OPTION LIST 8

Options

A Arrange chest X-ray, if results are normal then proceed
B Cancel the operation
C Defer operation and discuss at a multidisciplinary case conference
D Defer for 1 week
E Defer for 2 weeks
F Defer for 1 month
G Defer for 6 months
H Discharge woman, treat infection, readmit
I Discuss with anaesthetist
J Proceed on an emergency basis
K Proceed with the operation as planned
L Treat infection and defer the operation for 2 days

Instructions

The following clinical scenario refers to a woman who is scheduled to undergo surgery. However, you are asked to review the timing of the operation in the light of clinical circumstances described. Choose the **single** most appropriate management from the list of options for the item listed below.

Question

16 ▷ A 54-year-old woman with insulin-dependent diabetes has been admitted to undergo total abdominal hysterectomy and bilateral salpingo-oophorectomy for endometrial carcinoma. She was seen in the preoperative assessment clinic 5 days previously and the presence of an infected leg ulcer was noted. Methicillin-resistant *Staphylococcus aureus* was isolated by culture from a swab taken from the ulcer and you are shown the report after admission.

STEM/OPTION LIST 9

	Age (years)	Chief symptom(s)	Salient clinical and radiological findings	Clinical chemistry
A	18	Pelvic pain	Pelvic mass	Elevated serum αFP Elevated serum alpha-1 antitrypsin
B	18	Irregular vaginal bleeding Pelvic pain Blindness No history of recent pregnancy	Pelvic mass Intracranial space-occupying lesion	Elevated serum βhCG Normal serum αFP and CA125
C	14	Vaginal bleeding Precocious puberty	Pelvic mass	Elevated serum βhCG Elevated serum αFP
D	40	Postcoital bleeding	Necrotic mass in upper vagina Tumour-free space between lesion and pelvic sidewall No hydronephrosis	Normal serum αFP, βhCG, CA125

	Age (years)	Chief symptom(s)	Salient clinical and radiological findings	Clinical chemistry
E	50	Postcoital bleeding	Necrotic mass in upper vagina No tumour-free space between lesion and pelvic sidewall Unilateral hydronephrosis	Normal serum αFP, βhCG, CA125
F	60	Abdominal distension	Pelvic mass, ascites, stellate masses in omentum	Elevated serum CA125
G	40	Postcoital bleeding Sallow appearance	Pelvic mass with infiltration into the rectum Rectal ulceration Bilateral hydronephrosis	Normal serum CA125, αFP, βhCG
H	60		Bulky uterus with increased endometrial thickening	Normal serum CA125, αFP, HLG
I	52		Bulky uterus, increased endometrial thickening Unilateral adnexal mass with a diameter of 12 cm	Elevated serum inhibin. Serum FSH in the premenopausal range Normal serum CA125, αFP, βhCG
J	25	Irregular vaginal bleeding Early virilisation	Solid adnexal mass with a diameter of 6 cm	Elevated serum testosterone, normal serum CA125, αFP, βhCG

Instructions

For each of the following gynaecological malignancies, select the **single** most appropriate tumour profile from the list of options in the table above. Each option may be used once, more than once or not at all.

Questions

17 ▷ Stage 2 invasive cancer of the cervix.

18 ▷ Stage 3 invasive cancer of the cervix.

19 ▷ Stage 3 ovarian cancer.

STEM/OPTION LIST 10

Options

A	125.00	H	79.00
B	100.00	I	77.00
C	90.40	J	16.88
D	90.00	K	15.46
E	83.00	L	13.39
F	81.00	M	5.00
G	80.00	N	2.50

In a prospective blind study of a possible new method of antenatal fetal screening for a particular disorder, 5000 pregnant women rated as having a high risk for babies with this disorder were recruited and tested. These were the results:

	Baby born with disorder	**Baby born without disorder**	**Totals**
Tested positive	200	475	675
Tested negative	50	4275	4325
Totals	**250**	**4750**	**5000**

Instructions

For the item described below, choose the **single** most appropriate figure (rounded to two decimal points) from the above list.

Question

20 ▷ The prevalence of this disorder in this population.

STEM/OPTION LIST II

Options

- A Anticipate spontaneous vaginal delivery
- B Apply suprapubic pressure
- C Caesarean hysterectomy
- D Immediate caesarean section with myomectomy
- E Immediate lower-segment caesarean section
- F Immediate upper-segment caesarean section
- G Kjelland forceps delivery
- H Low enema
- I Lower-segment caesarean section within 30 minutes
- J Outlet forceps delivery
- K Upper-segment caesarean section within 30 minutes
- L Zavanelli manoeuvre

Instructions

The following clinical scenarios refer to an otherwise healthy 30-year-old pregnant woman who is in the second stage of labour in a modern and well-equipped labour ward. The woman's antenatal course was clinically uneventful and an ultrasound examination carried out at 19 weeks showed that the placenta was sited on the posterior uterine wall and was not low lying. Please choose the **single** most appropriate management for each scenario from the list of options. Each option may be used once, more than once or not at all.

Questions

21 ▷ The woman is a primigravida who was known to have a fundal fibroid with a diameter of 10 cm. At 40 weeks of gestation, spontaneous labour has developed. After a normal first stage lasting 6 hours and after the woman has been fully dilated for 30 minutes, the baby's head is crowning in the direct occipito-anterior position.

22 ▷ The woman is a primigravida who was known to have a fundal fibroid with a diameter of 10 cm. At 40 weeks of gestation, spontaneous labour has developed. After a normal first stage lasting 6 hours the cervix becomes fully dilated, the vertex is at the level of the spines and in the direct occipito-anterior position with minimal caput and moulding. No part of the head can be palpated per abdomen. The fetal heart rate suddenly drops to 65 beats/minute and the maternal pulse rate is 92 beats/minute and regular. After 5 minutes there is no recovery in the fetal heart rate.

23 ▷ The woman is a primigravida with a twin pregnancy. At a gestational age of 36 weeks, both twins are presenting by the vertex and spontaneous labour has developed. Following a first stage of 8 hours' duration, the woman becomes fully dilated and is draining liquor, which is thinly stained with meconium, and the cardiotocogram remains reassuring. On vaginal examination, you note that the left arm of the first twin has prolapsed into the vagina.

24 ▷ The woman is a primigravida with a twin pregnancy. At a gestational age of 36 weeks, both twins are presenting by the vertex and spontaneous labour has developed. Following a first stage of 8 hours' duration, the woman becomes fully dilated and is draining liquor, which is thinly stained with meconium, and cord prolapse occurs. The cord is pulsating.

25 ▷ The woman is 40 weeks into her second pregnancy and she has one living child aged 3 years who was delivered by elective lower-segment caesarean section for breech presentation. Following appropriate counselling, the woman has chosen to undergo vaginal delivery. Labour has started spontaneously. The first stage lasted 8 hours. Cartiotocography was reassuring and the amniotic fluid was noted to be clear. The woman had an epidural block and began to bear down after being in the second stage for 30 minutes. Delayed decelerations are noted in the cardiotocogram, the woman complains of increasing abdominal pain, there is a brisk trickle of blood per vaginam and the head is not clearly palpable in the pelvis on examination.

STEM/OPTION LIST 12

Options

A Amniotomy of the second twin's membranes
B Amniotomy of the second twin's membranes and intravenous oxytocin infusion
C Anticipate spontaneous vertex delivery
D Conservative management for at least 90 minutes
E Emergency caesarean section with De Lee's incision
F Emergency lower-segment caesarean section
G Emergency upper-segment caesarean section
H Encourage woman to deliver in knee-to-chest position
I Encourage woman to deliver in right lateral position
J Intravenous atosiban as a bolus
K Intravenous atosiban infusion
L Intravenous oxytocin infusion
M Intravenous syntometrine
N Outlet forceps delivery
O Subcutaneous terbutaline infusion
P Ultrasound assessment of the second twin's cardiac pulsations

Instructions

The following labour ward scenarios refer to an otherwise healthy 29-year-old primigravida who has received adequate antenatal care and who is in spontaneous labour with twins at a gestation of 38 weeks. Both twins were in longitudinal lie with vertex presentation when the woman was admitted to the labour ward. For each of the scenarios, choose the **single** most appropriate management from the list of options. Each option may be used once, more than once or not at all.

Questions

26 ▷ Following normal delivery of the first twin, you note that the uterine contractions are strong on palpation with a frequency of 1 in 2. The second twin has a longitudinal lie, the fetal heart rate tracing shows a single prolonged deceleration with good recovery and 5 minutes have elapsed since the delivery of the first twin. On vaginal examination, you note that the membranes of the second twin are bulging. The vertex appears to be just below the spines and you are unable to determine the position.

27 ▷ Following normal delivery of the first twin, you note that there is no uterine activity. The second twin has a longitudinal lie, the fetal heart rate tracing is reassuring and 15 minutes have elapsed since the delivery of the first twin. On vaginal examination, you note that the cervix is fully dilated, the membranes are bulging and the vertex is 1 cm below the spines.

28 ▷ Following delivery of the first twin, the membranes of the second twin rupture spontaneously. Cord prolapse occurs and you note on vaginal examination that the presenting part is above the level of the spines and you are unable to ascertain its position. The cord is pulsating slowly.

29 ▷ Following delivery of the first twin, the membranes of the second twin rupture spontaneously. On vaginal examination, cord prolapse is excluded but you note that an upper limb is in the vagina and one of the shoulders of the second twin can be palpated at the level of the spines.

STEM/OPTION LIST 13

Options

- A Administer betamethasone
- B Arrange abdominal X-ray
- C Arrange appropriate review in the antenatal clinic
- D Arrange CT pelvimetry
- E Check Kleihauer test prior to any procedure
- F Clinical pelvimetry
- G Elective lower-segment caesarean section at 39 weeks
- H Emergency lower-segment caesarean section
- I External cephalic version
- J External cephalic version under general anaesthesia
- K External cephalic version under spinal block
- L External cephalic version with inhalational analgesia
- M External cephalic version with oral mifepristone
- N External cephalic version with use of an appropriate myometrial relaxant
- O Induction of labour by forewater amniotomy
- P Induction of labour by insertion of prostaglandin E_2 vaginal gel

Instructions

The following scenarios refer to a pregnant woman aged 34 years, with a single fetus presenting by the breech. For each item, select the **single** most appropriate management from the list of options. Each option may be used once, more than once or not at all.

Questions

30 ▷ The woman is 38 weeks into her first pregnancy and her body mass index is 40.

31 ▷ The woman is 38 weeks into her second pregnancy and she has a healthy 2-year-old child who was delivered normally. There are no other obstetric or medical risk factors.

32 ▷ The woman is 28 weeks into her second pregnancy and she has a healthy 2-year-old child who was delivered normally. Breech presentation is noted in the antenatal clinic. There are no other obstetric or medical risk factors.

STEM/OPTION LIST 14

Options

A Serum Hb 12.1 g/dl, WCC 14×10^9/l, platelets 255×10^9/l, serum amylase 1200 iu/l , random serum glucose 10.7 mmol/l, no pathogenic organisms isolated by culture from MSU or high vaginal swab.

B Serum Hb 12.1 g/dl, WCC 11.5×10^9/l, platelets 255×10^9/l, serum amylase 50 iu/l, random serum glucose 6.7 mmol/l, sterile pyuria.

C Serum Hb 12.1 g/dl, WCC 13×10^9/l, platelets 255×10^9/l, serum amylase 50 iu/l, random serum glucose 6.7 mmol/l, Gram negative intracellular diplococci seen in material obtained from an endocervical swab.

D Serum Hb 12.1 g/dl, WCC 8×10^9/l, platelets 255×10^9/l, serum amylase 40 iu/l, random serum glucose 6.7 mmol/l, positive Sabin–Feldman dye test and corresponding IgM positive at a high titre.

E Serum Hb 12.1 g/dl, WCC 8×10^9/l, platelets 255×10^9/l, serum amylase 40 iu/l, random serum glucose 6.7 mmol/l, serum CA125 1200 iu/l, microscopic haematuria in MSU, no pathogenic organisms isolated by culture from MSU.

F Serum Hb 12.1 g/dl, WCC 8×10^9/l, platelets 255×10^9/l, serum amylase 40 iu/l, random serum glucose 6.7 mmol/l, serum CA125 55 iu/l, no pathogenic organisms isolated by culture from MSU.

G Serum Hb 12.1 g/dl, WCC 18×10^9/l, platelets 255×10^9/l, serum amylase 40 iu/l, random serum glucose 6.7 mmol/l, negative Sabin–Feldman dye test.

H Serum Hb 7.0 g/dl, WCC 1.8×10^9/l, platelets 55×10^9/l serum amylase 40 iu/l, random serum glucose 6.7 mmol/l, serum CA125 9 iu/l, no pathogenic organisms isolated by culture from MSU.

N Serum Hb 12.1g/dl, WCC 8×10^9/l, platelets 25×10^9/l, serum amylase 40iu/l, random serum glucose 6.7mmol/l, *Treponema pallidum* haemagglutination test positive at high titre, fluorescent treponemal antibody adsorption test strongly positive.

J Serum Hb 12.1g/dl, WCC 8×10^9/l, platelets 255×10^9/l, serum amylase 40iu/l, random serum glucose 6.7mmol/l, anticardiolipin IgG and IgM present in blood at a high titre.

K Serum Hb 12.1g/dl, WCC 14.5×10^9/l, platelets 255×10^9/l, serum amylase 50iu/l, random serum glucose 6.7mmol/l, significant growth of *Escherichia coli* isolated by culture from MSU.

L Serum Hb 12.1g/dl, WCC 14.5×10^9/l, platelets 255×10^9/l, serum amylase 50iu/l, random serum glucose 6.7mmol/l, significant growth of *Streptococcus faecalis* isolated by culture from MSU.

M Serum Hb 16.1g/dl, WCC 11.5×10^9/l, platelets 255×10^9/l, serum amylase 50iu/l, random serum glucose 6.7mmol/l.

N Serum Hb 12.1g/dl, WCC 13×10^9/l, platelets 255×10^9/l, serum amylase 50iu/l, random serum glucose 6.7mmol/l, clue cells seen on microscopic examination of material from a high vaginal swab.

Instructions

For each of the following women choose the **single** most likely set of laboratory findings from the list of options. Each option may be used once, more than once or not at all.

Questions

33 ▷ A 24-year-old primigravida complains of headache, fever and malaise at a gestation of 16 weeks. The salient finding on examination is generalised lymphadenopathy; the fetal condition appears satisfactory. The woman has been assisting her sister, who is a veterinary surgeon, and you are concerned that the diagnosis is acute maternal toxoplasmosis.

34 ▷ A 56-year-old woman attends your clinic as she has noticed increasing abdominal girth and epigastric discomfort. On examination, you note the presence of ascites and although a pelvic mass cannot be easily palpated you are concerned that the woman may have ovarian cancer.

35 ▷ A 36-year-old nulliparous woman complains of dyspareunia, dysmenorrhoea and menorrhagia. The salient finding on examination is tenderness in the posterior fornix of the vagina. You have discussed your findings with the woman and she has agreed to undergo diagnostic laparoscopy for investigation and to determine whether or not she has pelvic endometriosis.

STEM/OPTION LIST 15

Options

A Androgen-secreting adrenal tumour
B Androgen-secreting ovarian tumour
C Carcinoid syndrome
D Chronic liver failure
E Conn syndrome
F Cushing syndrome
G Ectopic ACTH production
H Hypothyroidism
I Idiopathic hirsutism
J Klinefelter syndrome
K Polycystic ovary syndrome
L Pure gonadal dysgenesis

Instructions

The following clinical scenarios refer to a non-pregnant woman who is very concerned by hirsutism. For each item, choose the **single** most likely diagnosis from the list of options. Each option may be used once, more than once or not at all.

Questions

36 ▷ The woman is aged 34 years and has a 12-month history of primary infertility and a long-standing history of oligomenorrhoea. She complains of hisutism. The results of her partner's semen analysis are normal. The serum testosterone is 3.5 nmol/l. Serum dehydroepiandrosterone sulphate, serum 17-α-hydroxyprogesterone and urinary free cortisol are well within their normal ranges.

37 ▷ The woman is aged 34 years. She complains of increased facial hair growth and has a 6-month history of oligomenorrhoea and a long-standing history of mild hypertension. She has recently noticed that she gets tired at work as a typist. Serum testosterone, serum dehydroepiandrosterone sulphate, serum 17-α-hydroxyprogesterone and serum urea and electrolytes are normal. The 24-hour urinary cortisol output is 1200 nmol/l with failure of suppression on low-dose dexamethasone (0.5 mg four times p.o.) but suppression on high-dose dexamethasone (2 mg four times p.o.)

38 ▷ The woman has mild hirsutism, with irregular and heavy menstrual bleeding. Ultrasound examination of the pelvis was incomplete, with poor visualisation of the ovaries, but increased endometrial thickness was noted. The uterus appeared to be normal. The serum LH was greater than serum FSH and the serum testosterone, serum dehydroepiandrosterone sulphate, serum 17-α-hydroxyprogesterone and serum urea and electrolytes were well within the normal range.

STEM/OPTION LIST 16

Options

A Absent P waves in the ECG
B Complete heart block
C Diminished P waves in the ECG
D Fall in oxygen saturation
E Fall in the respiratory rate

F Hypertension
G Hypotension
H Hypothermia (less than 36 degrees Celsius)
I Jugular venous engorgement
J Low-grade pyrexia (37.6 degrees Celsius)
K Progressive rise in temperature to 41 degrees Celsius
L Pulsus paradoxus
M Rising oxygen saturation
N Rising pulse rate and a normal respiratory rate
O Rising respiratory rate
P Sinus bradycardia

Instructions

Each of the following scenarios refers to a woman who has undergone major gynaecological surgery under general anaesthesia. The woman is now in the recovery area of the operation theatre. Other than the indication for the operation the woman has been healthy. For each of the scenarios, select the **single** most likely finding from the list of options. Each option may be used once, more than once or not at all.

Questions

39 ▷ The woman receives intravenous doxapram.

40 ▷ The woman develops acute and massive retention of urine due to a blocked urinary catheter.

5 | Mock examination 2

STEM OPTION LIST 1

Options

	Surface antigen	Antibodies to surface antigen	Hepatitis B DNA	Total core antibodies	'e' antigen	Antibodies to 'e' antigen
A	Negative	Positive	Negative	Negative	Negative	Negative
B	Positive	Positive	Negative	Negative	Negative	Negative
C	Positive	Negative	—	—	Negative	Positive
D	Negative	Negative	Negative	Negative	Negative	Positive
E	Positive	Negative	Positive	Negative	Positive	Negative
F	Negative	Positive	Negative	Positive	Negative	Positive
G	Negative	Negative	Negative	Negative	Negative	Negative
H	Negative	Negative	Positive	Positive	Positive	Negative
I	Negative	Positive	Negative	Negative	Positive	Negative
J	Negative	Negative	Negative	Positive	Positive	Negative

A pregnant woman has booked for antenatal care and undergoes serological tests for hepatitis B. For each of the following clinical conditions, choose from the list of options the item that shows the serological findings that would be expected. Each option may be used once, more than once or not at all.

Questions

1 ▷ Evidence of previous successful vaccination.

2 ▷ Evidence of carriage.

3 ▷ Evidence of carriage with a high risk of being infectious.

4 ▷ No evidence of infection.

5 ▷ The woman gives a history of vaccination against hepatitis B 6 months previously but the vaccine has been unsuccessful.

STEM/OPTION LIST 2

Options

A Anticipate spontaneous vaginal delivery
B Apply suprapubic pressure
C Caesarean hysterectomy
D Immediate caesarean section with myomectomy
E Immediate lower-segment caesarean section
F Immediate upper-segment caesarean section
G Kjelland forceps delivery
H Low enema
I Lower-segment caesarean section within 30 minutes
J Outlet forceps delivery
K Upper-segment caesarean section within 30 minutes
L Zavanelli manoeuvre

Instructions

The following clinical scenarios refer to an otherwise healthy 30-year-old pregnant woman who is in the second stage of labour in a modern and well-equipped labour ward. The woman's antenatal course was clinically uneventful and an ultrasound examination carried out at 19 weeks showed that the placenta was sited on the posterior uterine wall and not low lying. Choose the **single** most appropriate management for each scenario from the list of options. Each option may be used once, more than once or not at all.

Questions

6 ▷ The woman is a primigravida and has developed spontaneous labour at 38 weeks, the first stage lasting 6 hours. Intrapartum cardiotocography has been reassuring; liquor was clear. She has just become fully dilated with the vertex at a station of −1 and is now passing a large quantity of blood per vaginam. Although the maternal blood pressure remains at 100/60 mmHg, the woman's pulse rate has increased from 80 beats/minute to 110 beats/minute.

7 ▷ The woman is a primigravida and has developed spontaneous labour at 38 weeks, the first stage lasting 6 hours. Intrapartum cardiotocography has been reassuring and liquor was clear. She has just become fully dilated with the vertex at a station of −1 and cord prolapse occurs. On examination, you note that the cord is pulsating and the liquor is heavily stained with meconium.

8 ▷ The woman is 41 weeks into her first pregnancy. She has undergone induction of labour by insertion of prostaglandin vaginal gel, forewater amniotomy and intravenous oxytocin infusion. The first stage of labour lasted 11 hours. The woman has been receiving intravenous oxytocin infusion for 7 hours and an epidural block is in place. Two hours previously, full dilatation was noted. Active pushing commenced 1 hour ago and there is no progress. The cardiotocogram has been reassuring. On examination, you note that the vertex is at the level of the spines, one-fifth of the head is palpable per abdomen, the vertex is in the left occipito-lateral position, there is caput++ and a significant degree of moulding.

9 ▷ The woman is 40 weeks into her fourth pregnancy. She has three living children who were delivered normally. She has developed spontaneous labour. The first stage lasted 3 hours, full dilatation was noted 10 minutes ago and the head is crowning in the direct occipito-posterior position.

10 ▷ The woman is 34 weeks into her third pregnancy. She has two living children who were delivered by planned caesarean section at maternal request. She has just been admitted with regular contractions. The fetal heart rate tracing is satisfactory and the head is crowning in the direct occipito-anterior position.

STEM/OPTION LIST 3

Options

A Amniotomy of the second twin's membranes
B Amniotomy of the second twin's membranes and intravenous oxytocin infusion
C Anticipate spontaneous vertex delivery
D Conservative management for at least 90 minutes
E Emergency caesarean section with De Lee's incision
F Emergency lower-segment caesarean section
G Emergency upper-segment caesarean section
H Encourage woman to deliver in knee-to-chest position
I Encourage woman to deliver in right lateral position
J Intravenous atosiban as a bolus
K Intravenous atosiban infusion
L Intravenous oxytocin infusion
M Intravenous Syntometrine®
N Outlet forceps delivery
O Subcutaneous terbutaline infusion
P Ultrasound assessment of the second twin's cardiac pulsations

Instructions

The following labour ward scenarios refer to an otherwise healthy 29-year-old primigravida who has received adequate antenatal care and who is in spontaneous labour with twins at a gestation of 38 weeks. Both twins were in longitudinal lie with vertex presentation when the woman was admitted to the labour ward. For each of the scenarios, choose the **single** most appropriate management from the list of options. Each option may be used once, more than once or not at all.

Questions

11 ▷ The cervix has reached a dilatation of 8 cm after 5 hours of regular contractions. The vertex of the first twin is 1 cm below the spines and in the direct OA position. Both fetal heart rate tracings are reassuring. The woman is comfortable with an epidural block and is well supported by her partner.

12 ▷ The fetal heart rate tracing of the first twin shows bradycardia, with a fetal heart rate of 60 beats/minute over 10 minutes. On vaginal examination, you note that the cervix is fully dilated and the membranes are absent. The vertex is 1 cm below the spines and in the direct OA position.

13 ▷ Cord prolapse occurs at a cervical dilation of 8 cm. The vertex of the first twin is 1 cm above the spines and the fetal heart pulsations of the second twin are barely audible.

14 ▷ The fetal heart rate tracing of the first twin is reassuring but a satisfactory tracing of the heart rate of the second twin cannot be obtained using the abdominal transducer. On vaginal examination, you note that the cervix is 9 cm dilated and clear liquor is draining. The vertex of the first twin is at the level of the spines and in the OA position.

STEM/OPTION LIST 4

Options

A Administer betamethasone
B Arrange abdominal X-ray
C Arrange appropriate review in the antenatal clinic
D Arrange CT pelvimetry
E Check Kleihauer test prior to any procedure
F Clinical pelvimetry
G Elective lower-segment caesarean section at 39 weeks
H Emergency lower-segment caesarean section

I External cephalic version
J External cephalic version under general anaesthesia
K External cephalic version under spinal block
L External cephalic version with inhalational analgesia
M External cephalic version with oral mifepristone
N External cephalic version with use of an appropriate myometrial relaxant
O Induction of labour by forewater amniotomy
P Induction of labour by insertion of prostaglandin E_2 vaginal gel

Instructions

The following scenarios refer to a pregnant woman aged 34 years with a single fetus presenting by the breech. For each item, select the **single** most appropriate management from the list of options. Each option may be used once, more than once or not at all.

Questions

15 ▷ The woman is 38 weeks into her second pregnancy. She has one living child aged 3 years, who was delivered by emergency caesarean section for fetal distress. Other than the breech presentation, there are no other complications in the current pregnancy.

16 ▷ The woman is 38 weeks into her second pregnancy. She has one living child aged 3 years, who was delivered by emergency caesarean section for fetal distress. Other than the breech presentation, there are no other complications in the current pregnancy. The woman mentions that she is very hesitant to undergo blood transfusion.

17 ▷ The woman is 38 weeks into her first pregnancy. The pregnancy has been complicated by recurrent, mild, self-limiting antepartum haemorrhage of indeterminate origin.

STEM/OPTION LIST 5

Options

A Conservative management
B Elective caesarean section, ?ovarian cystectomy at 39 weeks
C Elective laparoscopy, ?proceed at 20 weeks of gestation
D Elective laparotomy at 10 weeks of gestation
E Elective laparotomy at 16 weeks of gestation
F Elective laparotomy at 28 weeks of gestation
G Elective laparotomy 6 weeks postnatally
H Emergency laparoscopy, ?proceed
I Emergency laparotomy
J Mini-laparotomy and ovarian biopsy

Instructions

The following clinical scenarios refer to an otherwise healthy 34-year-old pregnant woman who has booked for antenatal care. For each of the items listed below, choose the **single** most appropriate management from the list of options. Each option may be used once, more than once or not at all.

Questions

18 ▷ The woman is 12 weeks pregnant and she feels very well. The results of the booking scan show an ongoing intrauterine pregnancy with a single live fetus of 12 weeks' maturity. A simple left ovarian cyst is identified, with a diameter of 3.0 cm. There is no fluid in the pouch of Douglas.

19 ▷ The woman is 14 weeks pregnant and has been experiencing vague abdominal pain for several weeks. On clinical examination, the uterus is obviously large for dates. Ultrasound examination shows the presence of an ongoing intrauterine pregnancy with a single live fetus of 14 weeks' maturity. There is a right ovarian cyst, which is solid and homogenous; its diameter is 12 cm.

20 ▷ The woman is 11 weeks pregnant and complains of severe abdominal pain of 12 hours' duration. On examination, the woman is in obvious distress and there is tenderness on palpation of the abdomen. There is a pelvic mass and a neutrophil leucocytosis, with a total white cell count of 17.2×10^9/l. Ultrasound examination shows the presence of an ongoing intrauterine pregnancy, with a single live fetus of 11 weeks' maturity. There is a right adnexal mass with a diameter of 14 cm and free fluid in the pelvis.

21 ▷ The woman is 12 weeks pregnant and asymptomatic. There is a pelvic mass, which is almost reaching the umbilicus. Ultrasound examination shows the presence of an ongoing intrauterine twin pregnancy and each fetus has a maturity of 12 weeks. There is an ovarian cyst containing solid areas and the diameter of the lesion is 20 cm.

STEM/OPTION LIST 6

Options

- A Barrier contraception
- B Combined oral contraceptive pill
- C General advice on postcoital contraception only
- D Intrauterine contraceptive device
- E Laparoscopic tubal ligation
- F Laparotomy, tubal ligation
- G Long-acting injectable progestogen
- H Postcoital vaginal douche
- I Progestogen-only pill
- J Timed coitus

Instructions

The clinical scenarios listed below refer to a woman who has just undergone suction termination of pregnancy at 10 weeks of gestation, with no complications. In each situation, choose the **single** most appropriate form of contraception from the list of options. Each option may be used once, more than once or not at all.

Questions

22 ▷ The woman is aged 14 years, in good health, pleasant and has mild learning difficulties.

23 ▷ The woman is 40 years old, her serum has reacted positive to HIV and her relationship has ended.

24 ▷ The woman is 29 years old and in good health. She appears to be well motivated and has a history of menstrual irregularity.

25 ▷ The woman is 29 years old and in good health. She has one living child who was delivered normally. She has been pregnant four times in all, has undergone three induced abortions in total and is in a monogamous relationship.

STEM/OPTION LIST 7

Options

A Serum Hb 12.1 g/dl, WCC 14×10^9/l, platelets 255×10^9/l, serum amylase 1200 iu/l, random serum glucose 10.7 mmol/l, no pathogenic organisms isolated by culture from MSU or high vaginal swab.

B Serum Hb 12.1 g/dl, WCC 11.5×10^9/l, platelets 255×10^9/l, serum amylase 50 iu/l, random serum glucose 6.7 mmol/l, sterile pyuria.

C Serum Hb 12.1 g/dl, WCC 13×10^9/l, platelets 255×10^9/l, serum amylase 50 iu/l, random serum glucose 6.7 mmol/l, Gram negative intracellular diplococci seen in material obtained from an endocervical swab.

D Serum Hb 12.1 g/dl, WCC 8×10^9/l, platelets 255×10^9/l, serum amylase 40 iu/l, random serum glucose 6.7 mmol/l, positive Sabin–Feldman dye test and corresponding IgM positive at a high titre.

E Serum Hb 12.1 g/dl, WCC 8×10^9/l, platelets 255×10^9/l, serum amylase 40 iu/l, random serum glucose 6.7 mmol/l, serum CA125 1200 iu/l, microscopic haematuria in MSU, no pathogenic organisms isolated by culture from MSU.

F Serum Hb 12.1 g/dl, WCC 8×10^9/l, platelets 255×10^9/l, serum amylase 40 iu/l, random serum glucose 6.7 mmol/l, serum CA125 55 iu/l, no pathogenic organisms isolated by culture from MSU.

G Serum Hb 12.1 g/dl, WCC 18×10^9/l, platelets 255×10^9/l, serum amylase 40 iu/l, random serum glucose 6.7 mmol/l, negative Sabin–Feldman dye test.

H Serum Hb 7.0 g/dl, WCC 1.8×10^9/l, platelets 55×10^9/l, serum amylase 40 iu/l, random serum glucose 6.7 mmol/l, serum CA125 9 iu/l, no pathogenic organisms isolated by culture from MSU.

I Serum Hb 12.1 g/dl, WCC 8×10^9/l, platelets 255×10^9/l, serum amylase 40 iu/l, random serum glucose 6.7 mmol/l, *Treponema pallidum* haemagglutination test positive at high titre, fluorescent treponemal antibody adsorption test strongly positive.

J Serum Hb 12.1 g/dl, WCC 8×10^9/l, platelets 255×10^9/l, serum amylase 40 iu/l, random serum glucose 6.7 mmol/l, anticardiolipin IgG and IgM present in blood at a high titre.

K Serum Hb 12.1 g/dl, WCC 14.5×10^9/l, platelets 255×10^9/l, serum amylase 50 iu/l, random serum glucose 6.7 mmol/l, significant growth of *Escherichia coli* isolated by culture from MSU.

L Serum Hb 12.1 g/dl, WCC 14.5×10^9/l, platelets 255×10^9/l, serum amylase 50 iu/l, random serum glucose 6.7 mmol/l, significant growth of *Streptococcus faecalis* isolated by culture from MSU.

M Serum Hb 16.1 g/dl, WCC 11.5×109/l, platelets 255×109/l, serum amylase 50 iu/l, random serum glucose 6.7 mmol/l.

N Serum Hb 12.1 g/dl, WCC 13×10^9/l, platelets 255×10^9/l, serum amylase 50 iu/l, random serum glucose 6.7 mmol/l, clue cells seen on microscopic examination of material from a high vaginal swab.

Instructions

For each of the following women, choose the **single** most likely laboratory findings from the list of options. Each option may be used once, more than once or not at all.

Questions

26 ▷ A previously healthy 30-year-old primigravida is 29 weeks pregnant and is admitted with a history of epigastric pain of rapid onset. The salient features on examination are tachycardia and quiet bowel sounds. The fetal condition is satisfactory. You consider a diagnosis of acute pancreatitis.

27 ▷ A 22-year-old woman with a recent history of chlamydial infection of the cervix has been admitted with clinical features of mild pelvic inflammatory disease.

28 ▷ A 22-year-old woman had undergone investigations at the genito-urinary medicine clinic. She was found to have *Neisseria gonorrhoea* but she defaulted from follow up and treatment and is now admitted with clinical features of acute pelvic inflammatory disease.

STEM/OPTION LIST 8

Options

A Androgen-secreting adrenal tumour
B Androgen-secreting ovarian tumour
C Carcinoid syndrome
D Chronic liver failure
E Conn syndrome
F Cushing syndrome
G Ectopic ACTH production
H Hypothyroidism
I Idiopathic hirsutism
J Klinefelter syndrome

K Polycystic ovary syndrome
L Pure gonadal dysgenesis

Instructions

The following clinical scenarios refer to a non-pregnant woman who is very concerned by hirsutism. For each item, choose the **single** most likely diagnosis from the list of options. Each option may be used once, more than once or not at all.

Quesstions

29 ▷ The woman is aged 48 years and has noticed the growth of facial hair over the previous 6 months. She has been amenorrhoeic for the last 4 months; she has a deep voice and appears to have a fine tremor. The results of ultrasound examination of the pelvis are normal; the serum testosterone is 6 nmol/l; serum dehydroepiandrosterone sulphate is elevated; urinary free cortisol output is normal; serum 17-α-hydroxyprogesterone is well within the normal range and the serum FSH is greater than serum LH.

30 ▷ The woman is aged 24 years and is worried by hirsutism, which she says has developed rapidly over the last 3 months. She has noticed that her skin is more 'oily' and she has been amenorrhoeic for 2 months. Ultrasound examination of the pelvis shows the presence of a left adnexal mass with a diameter of 4 cm. The lesion is possibly part of the left ovary but the view is partly obscured by gas in the bowel. The right ovary is not visualised and the uterus is normal. The serum testosterone is 6 nmol/l, serum dehydroepiandrosterone sulphate, serum 17-α-hydroxyprogesterone and urinary free cortisol are well within their normal ranges. The serum FSH is greater than serum LH.

31 ▷ The woman is aged 34 years and she is annoyed by hair growth on her upper lip and chin. She reports a 12-month history of oligomenorrhoea, superimposed on a previous history of regular periods 'like clockwork'. The salient clinical features on examination include a body mass index of 32, blood pressure in the left arm of 170/100 mmHg in the sitting position and evidence of peripheral muscle weakness.

STEM/OPTION LIST 9

Options

A Amputation of the cervix
B Ball diathermy to cervix
C Cone biopsy under general anaesthesia
D Cryocautery to cervix
E Discharge without further follow-up
F Laser ablation of the transformation zone
G LLETZ
H Punch biopsy of the cervix and discussion at a multidisciplinary meeting
I Repeat colposcopy 1 year later
J Repeat colposcopy and cervical smear within 8 weeks
K Take a cervical smear only
L Wedge biopsy under general anaesthesia
M Wedge biopsy under local anaesthesia
N Wedge biosy under inhalational analgesia

Instructions

The following scenarios refer to a woman with an abnormal cervical smear. For each item, choose the **single** most appropriate management from the list of options. Each option may be used once, more than once or not at all.

Questions

32 ▷ The woman is 32 weeks into her fifth pregnancy and it has just been noticed that her cervical smear taken 5 months previously has shown mild dyskaryosis. Colposcopic examination shows the presence of warty changes involving most of the transformation zone.

The squamocolumnar junction can be visualised with confidence.

33 ▷ The woman is 24 weeks into her fifth pregnancy and it has just been noticed that her cervical smear taken 5 months previously has shown mild dyskaryosis. Colposcopic examination shows the presence of what appears to be an invasive lesion on the cervix.

34 ▷ The woman was 24 weeks into her fifth pregnancy when it was noticed that her cervical smear taken 5 months previously had shown mild dyskaryosis. Colposcopic examination showed the presence of warty changes involving most of the transformation zone. The squamocolumnar junction was visualised with confidence. Repeat colposcopic examination during pregnancy was carried out 6 weeks later (at 30 weeks of gestation) and the lesion had enlarged significantly.

35 ▷ A non-pregnant 30-year-old woman had previously undergone treatment for cervical intraepithelial neoplasia (CIN) and a follow-up cervical smear taken 4 months later showed moderate dyskaryosis. The woman underwent further colposcopy, with treatment, and high-grade CIN was diagnosed histologically. Four months later, a cervical smear was taken and the result showed mild dyskaryosis. Colposcopy shows the presence of a focal acetowhite lesion in the transformation zone. The squamocolumnar junction can be visualised with confidence.

36 ▷ The woman is not pregnant. She is aged 50 years and the result of the cervical smear shows severe dyskaryosis. Colposcopic examination of the cervix is inconclusive.

37 ▷ The woman is not pregnant. She is aged 50 years; there is no history of menstrual irregularity and the result of the cervical smear shows glandular atypia. Colposcopic examination shows the presence of a small lesion with some of the features of adenocarcinoma.

STEM/OPTION LIST 10

Options

- A Absent P waves in the ECG
- B Complete heart block
- C Diminished P waves in the ECG
- D Fall in oxygen saturation
- E Fall in the respiratory rate
- F Hypertension
- G Hypotension
- H Hypothermia (less than 36 degrees Celsius)
- I Jugular venous engorgement
- J Low-grade pyrexia (37.6 degrees Celsius)
- K Progressive rise in temperature to 41 degrees Celsius
- L Pulsus paradoxus
- M Rising oxygen saturation
- N Rising pulse rate and a normal respiratory rate
- O Rising respiratory rate
- P Sinus bradycardia

Instructions

Each of the following scenarios refers to a woman who has undergone major gynaecological surgery under general anaesthesia. The woman is now in the recovery area of the operation theatre. Other than the indication for the operation, the woman has been healthy. For each of the scenarios, select the **single** most likely finding from the list of options. Each option may be used once, more than once or not at all.

Questions

38 ▷ The woman has undergone prolonged abdominal surgery with adequate haemostasis.

39 ▷ The woman receives an excessive dose of neostigmine for reversal of muscle relaxation.

40 ▷ There is obstruction of the airway.

6 | Mock examination 1 answers

STEM/OPTION LIST 1

Theme ▷ Obstetrics and gynaecology: drug usages, mode of administration.

Domain ▷ Management.

Answers

1 ▶ *D* = Continuous intravenous infusion.

2 ▶ *J* = Intravenous injection.

3 ▶ *L* = Per oram.

4 ▶ *J* = Intravenous injection.

Notes on answers

For worked examples covering this option list, see the Stem/option list 2 in Chapter 3 and its commentary.

STEM/OPTION LIST 2

Theme ▷ Obstetrics: maternal infection, toxoplasmosis.

Domain ▷ Diagnosis.

Answers

5 ▶ *C* = Acute maternal toxoplasmosis.

6 ▶ *C* = Acute maternal toxoplasmosis.

Notes on answers

For worked examples covering this option list, see the Stem/option list 4 in Chapter 3 and its commentary.

STEM/OPTION LIST 3

Theme ▷ Obstetrics: prepregnancy, antenatal counselling, congenital adrenal hyperplasia.

Domain ▷ Genetics.

Answer

7 ▶ *I* = 1 in 8.

Notes on answer

For worked examples covering this option list, see the Stem/option list 5 in Chapter 3 and its commentary. This item is a parallel to *Item 2* of the worked example. The risk of an affected daughter is the same as the risk of an affected son and thus is 1 in 4 × 1 in 2 = 1 in 8. Therefore, the answer is *I*.

STEM/OPTION LIST 4

Theme ▷ Obstetrics: prepregnancy, antenatal counselling.

Domain ▷ Genetics: X-linked dominance.

Answer

8 ▶ *K* = 1 in 2.

Notes on answer

For worked examples covering this option list, see the Stem/option list 6 in Chapter 3 and its commentary. Note that, if the baby is affected in this pregnancy then the risk of having an affected child in the next pregnancy would still be 1 in 2.

STEM/OPTION LIST 5

Theme ▷ Obstetrics: prenatal diagnosis of Down syndrome.

Domain ▷ Diagnosis, investigations.

Answers

9 ▶ *B*=Amniocentesis at 16 weeks for karyotype.

10 ▶ *I*=No further action.

Notes on answers

For worked examples covering this option list, see the Stem/option list 8 in Chapter 3 and its commentary.

Item 9=B ▶ This 38-year-old primigravida, at a gestational age of 13 weeks, has a significant age-related risk of having a child with Down syndrome. Therefore, the answer is *B*.

Item 10=I ▶ This woman has a low risk of having a child with Down syndrome and therefore, the answer is *I*.

STEM/OPTION LIST 6

Theme ▷ Gynaecology: perimenopausal contraception.

Domain ▷ Management.

Answers

11 ▷ *O*=Stop using contraception.

12 ▷ *O*=Stop using contraception.

Notes on answers

For worked examples covering this option list, see the Stem/option list 9 in Chapter 3 and its commentary.

STEM/OPTION LIST 7

Theme ▷ Gynaecology: contraception, progestogen-based.

Domain ▷ Pharmacology: prescribing administration, management.

Answers

13 ▶ *B*=Once daily.

14 ▶ *L*=Once every 12 weeks.

15 ▶ *L*=Once every 12 weeks.

Notes on answers

For worked examples covering this option list, see the Stem/option list 10 in Chapter 3 and its commentary. Norethisterone refers to a different formulation of progestogen-only pills (like the worked examples 1 and 2). Therefore, the answer to *Item 13* is *A*.

The concurrent use of pharmacological agents that induce liver enzymes does not appear to affect the efficacy of medroxyprogesterone acetate aqueous suspension. Therefore, the frequency of administration of medroxyprogesterone acetate aqueous suspension need not be altered for women taking carbamazepine. Hence, the answer to *Item 5* is also *L*.

STEM/OPTION LIST 8

Theme ▷ Gynaecology: surgery.

Domain ▷ Clinical prioritisation: management.

Answer

16 ▶ *H*=Discharge woman, treat infection, readmit.

Notes on answers

For worked examples covering this option list, see the Stem/option list 12 in Chapter 3 and its commentary. This 54-year-old woman, who has insulin-dependent diabetes, is to undergo transabdominal hysterectomy and bilateral salpingo-oorphorectomy for endometrial carcinoma. MRSA has been isolated from a leg ulcer. Despite the unquestionably high priority for carrying out the operation, it is best to treat the infection and defer the operation. Therefore, the answer is *H*.

STEM/OPTION LIST 9

Theme ▷ Gynaecology: oncology

Domain ▷ Diagnosis

Answers

17 ▶ *D*=40 years. Postcoital bleeding, necrotic mass in upper vagina. Tumour-free space between lesion and pelvic sidewall. No hydronephrosis. Normal serum αFP, βhCG, CA125.

18 ▶ *E*=50 years. Postcoital bleeding. Necrotic mass in upper vagina. No tumour-free space between lesion and pelvic sidewall. Unilateral hydronephrosis. Normal serum αFP, βhCG, CA125.

19 ▶ *F* = 60 years. Abdominal distension. Pelvic mass, ascites, stellate masses in omentum. Elevated serum CA125.

Notes on answers

For worked examples covering this option list, see the Stem/option list 13 in Chapter 3 and its commentary.

STEM/OPTION LIST 10

Theme ▷ Research methodology, antenatal screening.

Domain ▷ Statistics.

Answer

20 ▶ *M* = 5.00.

Notes on answers

For worked examples covering this option list, see the Stem/option list 14 in Chapter 3 and its commentary. This is another relatively simple calculation, as long as you know the definition. In this case, it is the number of babies born with the disorder (200) divided by the total population (5000).

STEM/OPTION LIST 11

Theme ▷ Obstetrics: second stage of labour.

Domain ▷ Management.

Answers

21 ▶ *A* = Anticipate spontaneous vaginal delivery.

22 ▶ *J* = Outlet forceps delivery.

23 ▶ *I* = Lower-segment caesarean section within 30 minutes.

24 ▶ *E* = Immediate lower-segment caesarean section.

25 ▶ *E* = Immediate lower-segment caesarean section.

STEM/OPTION LIST 12

Theme ▷ Obstetrics: twin pregnancy, management in labour.

Domain ▷ Management.

Answers

26 ▶ *A* = Amniotomy of the second twin's membranes.

27 ▶ *B* = Amniotomy of the second twin's membranes and intravenous oxytocin infusion.

28 ▶ *F* = Emergency lower-segment caesarean section.

29 ▶ *F* = Emergency lower-segment caesarean section.

STEM/OPTION LIST 13

Theme ▷ Obstetrics: breech presentation, external cephalic version.

Domain ▷ Management.

Answers

30 ▶ *G* = Elective lower-segment caesarean section at 39 weeks.

31 ▶ *N* = External cephalic version with use of an appropriate myometrial relaxant.

32 ▶ *C* = Arrange appropriate review in the antenatal clinic.

STEM/OPTION LIST 14

Theme ▷ Gynaecology: test results.

Domain ▷ Diagnosis.

Answers

33 ▶ *D*=Serum Hb 12.1 g/dl, WCC 8×10^9/l, platelets 255×10^9/l, serum amylase 40 iu/l, random serum glucose 6.7 mmol/l, positive Sabin-Feldman dye test and corresponding IgM positive at a high titre.

34 ▶ *E*=Serum Hb 12.1 g/dl, WCC 8×10^9/l, platelets 255×10^9/l, serum amylase 40 iu/l, random serum glucose 6.7 mmol/l, serum CA125 1200 iu/l, microscopic haematuria in MSU, no pathogenic organisms isolated by culture from MSU.

35 ▶ *F*=Serum Hb 12.1 g/dl, WCC 8×10^9/l, platelets 255×10^9/l, serum amylase 40 iu/l, random serum glucose 6.7 mmol/l, serum CA125 55 iu/l, no pathogenic organisms isolated by culture from MSU.

STEM/OPTION LIST 15

Theme ▷ Gynaecology: endocrinology, hirsutism.

Domain ▷ Diagnosis.

Answers

36 ▶ *K*=Polycystic ovary syndrome.

37 ▶ *F*=Cushing syndrome.

38 ▶ *K*=Polycystic ovary syndrome.

STEM/OPTION LIST 16

Theme ▷ Gynaecology: postoperative complications (anaesthesia related).

Domain ▷ Diagnosis.

Answers

39 ▶ *O*=Rising respiratory rate.

40 ▶ *F*=Hypertension.

7 | Mock examination 2 answers

STEM/OPTION LIST 1

Theme ▷ Obstetrics.

Domain ▷ Hepatitis B serology, antenatal care.

Answers

1 ▶ *A* = Surface antigen (Negative). Antibodies to surface antigen (Positive). Hepatitis B DNA (Negative). Total core antibodies (Negative). 'e' antigen (Negative). Antibodies to 'e' antigen (Negative).

2 ▶ *C* = Surface antigen (Positive). Antibodies to surface antigen (Negative). Hepatitis D DNA (–). Total core antibodies (–). 'e' antigen (Negative). Antibodies to 'e' antigen (Positive).

3 ▶ *E* = Surface antigen (Positive). Antibodies to surface antigen (Negative). Hepatitis B DNA (Positive). Total core antibodies (Negative). 'e' antigen (Positive). Antibodies to 'e' antigen (Negative).

4 ▶ *G* = Surface antigen (Negative). Antibodies to surface antigen (Negative). Hepatitis B DNA (Negative). Total core antibodies (Negative). 'e' antigen (Negative). Antibodies to 'e' antigen (Negative).

5 ▶ *G* = Surface antigen (Negative). Antibodies to surface antigen (Negative). Hepatitis B DNA (Negative). Total core antibodies (Negative). 'e' antigen (Negative). Antibodies to 'e' antigen (Negative).

STEM/OPTION LIST 2

Theme ▷ Obstetrics: second stage of labour.

Domain ▷ Management.

Answers

6 ▶ *E* = Immediate lower-segment caesarean section.

7 ▶ *E* = Immediate lower-segment caesarean section.

8 ▶ *I* = Lower-segment caesarean section within 30 minutes.

9 ▶ *A* = Anticipate spontaneous vaginal delivery.

10 ▶ *A* = Anticipate spontaneous vaginal delivery.

STEM/OPTION LIST 3

Theme ▷ Obstetrics: twin pregnancy, management in labour.

Domain ▷ Management.

Answers

11 ▶ *C* = Anticipate spontaneous vertex delivery.

12 ▶ *N* = Outlet forceps delivery.

13 ▶ *F* = Emergency lower-segment caesarean section.

14 ▶ *P* = Ultrasound assessment of the second twin's cardiac pulsations.

STEM/OPTION LIST 4

Theme ▷ Obstetrics: breech presentation, external cephalic version.

Domain ▷ Management.

Answers

15 ▶ *G* = Elective lower-segment caesarean section at 39 weeks.

16 ▶ *G* = Elective lower-segment caesarean section at 39 weeks.

17 ▶ *G* = Elective lower-segment caesarean section at 39 weeks.

STEM/OPTION LIST 5

Theme ▷ Obstetrics: ovarian cyst during pregnancy.

Domain ▷ Management.

18 ▶ *A* = Conservative management.

19 ▶ *E* = Elective laparotomy at 16 weeks of gestation.

20 ▶ *I* = Emergency laparotomy.

21 ▶ *E* = Elective laparotomy at 16 weeks of gestation.

STEM/OPTION LIST 6

Theme ▷ Gynaecology: post-pregnancy contraception.

Domain ▷ Management: pharmacology, administration.

Answers

22 ▶ *G* = Long-acting injectable progestogen. ? – 14.

23 ▶ *A* = Barrier contraception.

24 ▶ *B* = Combined oral contraceptive pill.

25 ▶ *D* = Intrauterine contraceptive device.

STEM/OPTION LIST 7

Theme ▷ Gynaecology: test results.

Domain ▷ Diagnosis.

Answers

26 ▶ *A* – Serum Hb 12.1 g/dl, WCC 14×10^9/l, platelets 255×10^9/l, serum amylase 1200 iu/l , random serum glucose 10.7 mmol/l, no pathogenic organisms isolated by culture from MSU or high vaginal swab.

27 ▶ *B* – Serum Hb 12.1 g/dl, WCC 11.5×10^9/l, platelets 255×10^9/l, serum amylase 50 iu/l, random serum glucose 6.7 mmol/l, sterile pyuria.

28 ▶ *C* – Serum Hb 12.1 g/dl, WCC 13×10^9/l, platelets 255×10^9/l, serum amylase 50 iu/l, random serum glucose 6.7 mmol/l, Gram negative intracellular diplococci seen in material obtained from an endocervical swab.

STEM/OPTION LIST 8

Theme ▷ Gynaecology: endocrinology, hirsutism.

Domain ▷ Diagnosis.

Answers

29 ▶ *A* = Androgen-secreting adrenal tumour.

30 ▶ *B* = Androgen-secreting ovarian tumour.

31 ▶ *F* = Cushing syndrome.

STEM/OPTION LIST 9

Theme ▷ Gynaecology: colposcopy, pregnant and nonpregnant.

Domain ▷ Management: surgical skills.

Answers

32 ▶ *K*=Take a cervical smear only.

33 ▶ *L*=Wedge biopsy under general anaesthesia.

34 ▶ *L*=Wedge biopsy under general anaesthesia.

35 ▶ *G*=LLETZ.

36 ▶ *C*=Cone biopsy under general anaesthesia.

37 ▶ *C*=Cone biopsy under general anaesthesia.

STEM/OPTION LIST 16

Theme ▷ Gynaecology: Postoperative complications (anaesthesia related).

Domain ▷ Diagnosis.

Answers

38 ▶ *H*=Hypothermia (less than 36 degrees Celsius).

39 ▶ *P*=Sinus bradycardia.

40 ▶ *D*=Fall in oxygen saturation.

Mock examination answer keys

Use these keys to quickly mark your self-testing efforts.

Mock examination 1

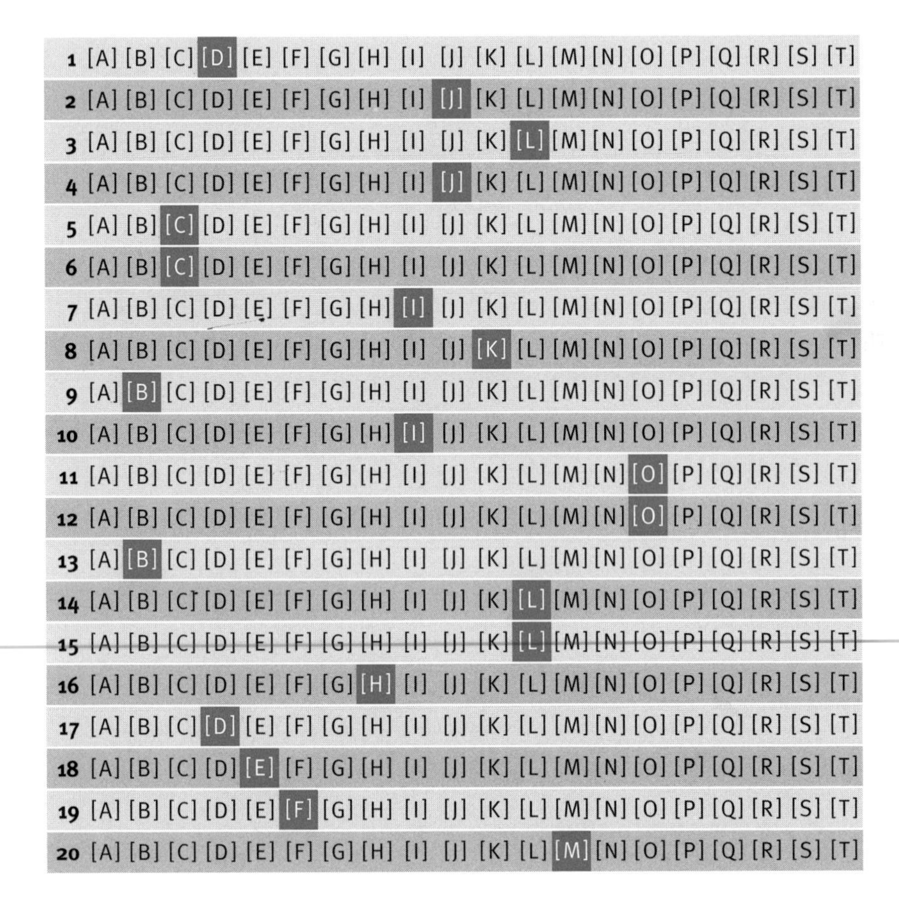

1 [A] [B] [C] **[D]** [E] [F] [G] [H] [I] [J] [K] [L] [M] [N] [O] [P] [Q] [R] [S] [T]
2 [A] [B] [C] [D] [E] [F] [G] [H] [I] **[J]** [K] [L] [M] [N] [O] [P] [Q] [R] [S] [T]
3 [A] [B] [C] [D] [E] [F] [G] [H] [I] [J] [K] **[L]** [M] [N] [O] [P] [Q] [R] [S] [T]
4 [A] [B] [C] [D] [E] [F] [G] [H] [I] **[J]** [K] [L] [M] [N] [O] [P] [Q] [R] [S] [T]
5 [A] [B] **[C]** [D] [E] [F] [G] [H] [I] [J] [K] [L] [M] [N] [O] [P] [Q] [R] [S] [T]
6 [A] [B] **[C]** [D] [E] [F] [G] [H] [I] [J] [K] [L] [M] [N] [O] [P] [Q] [R] [S] [T]
7 [A] [B] [C] [D] [E] [F] [G] [H] **[I]** [J] [K] [L] [M] [N] [O] [P] [Q] [R] [S] [T]
8 [A] [B] [C] [D] [E] [F] [G] [H] [I] [J] **[K]** [L] [M] [N] [O] [P] [Q] [R] [S] [T]
9 [A] **[B]** [C] [D] [E] [F] [G] [H] [I] [J] [K] [L] [M] [N] [O] [P] [Q] [R] [S] [T]
10 [A] [B] [C] [D] [E] [F] [G] [H] **[I]** [J] [K] [L] [M] [N] [O] [P] [Q] [R] [S] [T]
11 [A] [B] [C] [D] [E] [F] [G] [H] [I] [J] [K] [L] [M] [N] **[O]** [P] [Q] [R] [S] [T]
12 [A] [B] [C] [D] [E] [F] [G] [H] [I] [J] [K] [L] [M] [N] **[O]** [P] [Q] [R] [S] [T]
13 [A] **[B]** [C] [D] [E] [F] [G] [H] [I] [J] [K] [L] [M] [N] [O] [P] [Q] [R] [S] [T]
14 [A] [B] [C] [D] [E] [F] [G] [H] [I] [J] [K] **[L]** [M] [N] [O] [P] [Q] [R] [S] [T]
15 [A] [B] [C] [D] [E] [F] [G] [H] [I] [J] [K] **[L]** [M] [N] [O] [P] [Q] [R] [S] [T]
16 [A] [B] [C] [D] [E] [F] [G] **[H]** [I] [J] [K] [L] [M] [N] [O] [P] [Q] [R] [S] [T]
17 [A] [B] [C] **[D]** [E] [F] [G] [H] [I] [J] [K] [L] [M] [N] [O] [P] [Q] [R] [S] [T]
18 [A] [B] [C] [D] **[E]** [F] [G] [H] [I] [J] [K] [L] [M] [N] [O] [P] [Q] [R] [S] [T]
19 [A] [B] [C] [D] [E] **[F]** [G] [H] [I] [J] [K] [L] [M] [N] [O] [P] [Q] [R] [S] [T]
20 [A] [B] [C] [D] [E] [F] [G] [H] [I] [J] [K] [L] **[M]** [N] [O] [P] [Q] [R] [S] [T]

21 **[A]** [B] [C] [D] [E] [F] [G] [H] [I] [J] [K] [L] [M] [N] [O] [P] [Q] [R] [S] [T]
22 [A] [B] [C] [D] [E] [F] [G] [H] [I] **[J]** [K] [L] [M] [N] [O] [P] [Q] [R] [S] [T]
23 [A] [B] [C] [D] [E] [F] [G] [H] **[I]** [J] [K] [L] [M] [N] [O] [P] [Q] [R] [S] [T]
24 [A] [B] [C] [D] **[E]** [F] [G] [H] [I] [J] [K] [L] [M] [N] [O] [P] [Q] [R] [S] [T]
25 [A] [B] [C] [D] **[E]** [F] [G] [H] [I] [J] [K] [L] [M] [N] [O] [P] [Q] [R] [S] [T]
26 **[A]** [B] [C] [D] [E] [F] [G] [H] [I] [J] [K] [L] [M] [N] [O] [P] [Q] [R] [S] [T]
27 [A] **[B]** [C] [D] [E] [F] [G] [H] [I] [J] [K] [L] [M] [N] [O] [P] [Q] [R] [S] [T]
28 [A] [B] [C] [D] [E] **[F]** [G] [H] [I] [J] [K] [L] [M] [N] [O] [P] [Q] [R] [S] [T]
29 [A] [B] [C] [D] [E] **[F]** [G] [H] [I] [J] [K] [L] [M] [N] [O] [P] [Q] [R] [S] [T]
30 [A] [B] [C] [D] [E] [F] **[G]** [H] [I] [J] [K] [L] [M] [N] [O] [P] [Q] [R] [S] [T]
31 [A] [B] [C] [D] [E] [F] [G] [H] [I] [J] [K] [L] [M] **[N]** [O] [P] [Q] [R] [S] [T]
32 [A] [B] **[C]** [D] [E] [F] [G] [H] [I] [J] [K] [L] [M] [N] [O] [P] [Q] [R] [S] [T]
33 [A] [B] [C] **[D]** [E] [F] [G] [H] [I] [J] [K] [L] [M] [N] [O] [P] [Q] [R] [S] [T]
34 [A] [B] [C] [D] **[E]** [F] [G] [H] [I] [J] [K] [L] [M] [N] [O] [P] [Q] [R] [S] [T]
35 [A] [B] [C] [D] [E] **[F]** [G] [H] [I] [J] [K] [L] [M] [N] [O] [P] [Q] [R] [S] [T]
36 [A] [B] [C] [D] [E] [F] [G] [H] [I] [J] **[K]** [L] [M] [N] [O] [P] [Q] [R] [S] [T]
37 [A] [B] [C] [D] [E] **[F]** [G] [H] [I] [J] [K] [L] [M] [N] [O] [P] [Q] [R] [S] [T]
38 [A] [B] [C] [D] [E] [F] [G] [H] [I] [J] **[K]** [L] [M] [N] [O] [P] [Q] [R] [S] [T]
39 [A] [B] [C] [D] [E] [F] [G] [H] [I] [J] [K] [L] [M] [N] **[O]** [P] [Q] [R] [S] [T]
40 [A] [B] [C] [D] [E] **[F]** [G] [H] [I] [J] [K] [L] [M] [N] [O] [P] [Q] [R] [S] [T]

Mock examination 2

1	**[A]**	[B]	[C]	[D]	[E]	[F]	[G]	[H]	[I]	[J]	[K]	[L]	[M]	[N]	[O]	[P]	[Q]	[R]	[S]	[T]
2	[A]	[B]	**[C]**	[D]	[E]	[F]	[G]	[H]	[I]	[J]	[K]	[L]	[M]	[N]	[O]	[P]	[Q]	[R]	[S]	[T]
3	[A]	[B]	[C]	[D]	**[E]**	[F]	[G]	[H]	[I]	[J]	[K]	[L]	[M]	[N]	[O]	[P]	[Q]	[R]	[S]	[T]
4	[A]	[B]	[C]	[D]	[E]	[F]	**[G]**	[H]	[I]	[J]	[K]	[L]	[M]	[N]	[O]	[P]	[Q]	[R]	[S]	[T]
5	[A]	[B]	[C]	[D]	[E]	[F]	**[G]**	[H]	[I]	[J]	[K]	[L]	[M]	[N]	[O]	[P]	[Q]	[R]	[S]	[T]
6	[A]	[B]	[C]	[D]	**[E]**	[F]	[G]	[H]	[I]	[J]	[K]	[L]	[M]	[N]	[O]	[P]	[Q]	[R]	[S]	[T]
7	[A]	[B]	[C]	[D]	**[E]**	[F]	[G]	[H]	[I]	[J]	[K]	[L]	[M]	[N]	[O]	[P]	[Q]	[R]	[S]	[T]
8	[A]	[B]	[C]	[D]	[E]	[F]	[G]	[H]	**[I]**	[J]	[K]	[L]	[M]	[N]	[O]	[P]	[Q]	[R]	[S]	[T]
9	**[A]**	[B]	[C]	[D]	[E]	[F]	[G]	[H]	[I]	[J]	[K]	[L]	[M]	[N]	[O]	[P]	[Q]	[R]	[S]	[T]
10	**[A]**	[B]	[C]	[D]	[E]	[F]	[G]	[H]	[I]	[J]	[K]	[L]	[M]	[N]	[O]	[P]	[Q]	[R]	[S]	[T]
11	[A]	[B]	**[C]**	[D]	[E]	[F]	[G]	[H]	[I]	[J]	[K]	[L]	[M]	[N]	[O]	[P]	[Q]	[R]	[S]	[T]
12	[A]	[B]	[C]	[D]	[E]	[F]	[G]	[H]	[I]	[J]	[K]	[L]	[M]	**[N]**	[O]	[P]	[Q]	[R]	[S]	[T]
13	[A]	[B]	[C]	[D]	[E]	**[F]**	[G]	[H]	[I]	[J]	[K]	[L]	[M]	[N]	[O]	[P]	[Q]	[R]	[S]	[T]
14	[A]	[B]	[C]	[D]	[E]	[F]	[G]	[H]	[I]	[J]	[K]	[L]	[M]	[N]	[O]	**[P]**	[Q]	[R]	[S]	[T]
15	[A]	[B]	[C]	[D]	[E]	[F]	**[G]**	[H]	[I]	[J]	[K]	[L]	[M]	[N]	[O]	[P]	[Q]	[R]	[S]	[T]
16	[A]	[B]	[C]	[D]	[E]	[F]	**[G]**	[H]	[I]	[J]	[K]	[L]	[M]	[N]	[O]	[P]	[Q]	[R]	[S]	[T]
17	[A]	[B]	[C]	[D]	[E]	[F]	**[G]**	[H]	[I]	[J]	[K]	[L]	[M]	[N]	[O]	[P]	[Q]	[R]	[S]	[T]
18	**[A]**	[B]	[C]	[D]	[E]	[F]	[G]	[H]	[I]	[J]	[K]	[L]	[M]	[N]	[O]	[P]	[Q]	[R]	[S]	[T]
19	[A]	[B]	[C]	[D]	**[E]**	[F]	[G]	[H]	[I]	[J]	[K]	[L]	[M]	[N]	[O]	[P]	[Q]	[R]	[S]	[T]
20	[A]	[B]	[C]	[D]	[E]	[F]	[G]	[H]	**[I]**	[J]	[K]	[L]	[M]	[N]	[O]	[P]	[Q]	[R]	[S]	[T]

21 [A] [B] [C] [D] **[E]** [F] [G] [H] [I] [J] [K] [L] [M] [N] [O] [P] [Q] [R] [S] [T]

22 [A] [B] [C] [D] [E] [F] **[G]** [H] [I] [J] [K] [L] [M] [N] [O] [P] [Q] [R] [S] [T]

23 **[A]** [B] [C] [D] [E] [F] [G] [H] [I] [J] [K] [L] [M] [N] [O] [P] [Q] [R] [S] [T]

24 [A] **[B]** [C] [D] [E] [F] [G] [H] [I] [J] [K] [L] [M] [N] [O] [P] [Q] [R] [S] [T]

25 [A] [B] [C] **[D]** [E] [F] [G] [H] [I] [J] [K] [L] [M] [N] [O] [P] [Q] [R] [S] [T]

26 **[A]** [B] [C] [D] [E] [F] [G] [H] [I] [J] [K] [L] [M] [N] [O] [P] [Q] [R] [S] [T]

27 [A] **[B]** [C] [D] [E] [F] [G] [H] [I] [J] [K] [L] [M] [N] [O] [P] [Q] [R] [S] [T]

28 [A] [B] **[C]** [D] [E] [F] [G] [H] [I] [J] [K] [L] [M] [N] [O] [P] [Q] [R] [S] [T]

29 **[A]** [B] [C] [D] [E] [F] [G] [H] [I] [J] [K] [L] [M] [N] [O] [P] [Q] [R] [S] [T]

30 [A] **[B]** [C] [D] [E] [F] [G] [H] [I] [J] [K] [L] [M] [N] [O] [P] [Q] [R] [S] [T]

31 [A] [B] [C] [D] [E] **[F]** [G] [H] [I] [J] [K] [L] [M] [N] [O] [P] [Q] [R] [S] [T]

32 [A] [B] [C] [D] [E] [F] [G] [H] [I] [J] **[K]** [L] [M] [N] [O] [P] [Q] [R] [S] [T]

33 [A] [B] [C] [D] [E] [F] [G] [H] [I] [J] [K] **[L]** [M] [N] [O] [P] [Q] [R] [S] [T]

34 [A] [B] [C] [D] [E] [F] [G] [H] [I] [J] [K] **[L]** [M] [N] [O] [P] [Q] [R] [S] [T]

35 [A] [B] [C] [D] [E] [F] **[G]** [H] [I] [J] [K] [L] [M] [N] [O] [P] [Q] [R] [S] [T]

36 [A] [B] **[C]** [D] [E] [F] [G] [H] [I] [J] [K] [L] [M] [N] [O] [P] [Q] [R] [S] [T]

37 [A] [B] **[C]** [D] [E] [F] [G] [H] [I] [J] [K] [L] [M] [N] [O] [P] [Q] [R] [S] [T]

38 [A] [B] [C] [D] [E] [F] [G] **[H]** [I] [J] [K] [L] [M] [N] [O] [P] [Q] [R] [S] [T]

39 [A] [B] [C] [D] [E] [F] [G] [H] [I] [J] [K] [L] [M] [N] [O] **[P]** [Q] [R] [S] [T]

40 [A] [B] [C] **[D]** [E] [F] [G] [H] [I] [J] [K] [L] [M] [N] [O] [P] [Q] [R] [S] [T]

1 [A] [B] [C] [D] [E] [F] [G] [H] [I] [J] [K] [L] [M] [N] [O] [P] [Q] [R] [S] [T]

2 [A] [B] [C] [D] [E] [F] [G] [H] [I] [J] [K] [L] [M] [N] [O] [P] [Q] [R] [S] [T]

3	[A]	[B]	[C]	[D]	[E]	[F]	[G]	[H]	[I]	[J]	[K]	[L]	[M]	[N]	[O]	[P]	[Q]	[R]	[S]	[T]
4	[A]	[B]	[C]	[D]	[E]	[F]	[G]	[H]	[I]	[J]	[K]	[L]	[M]	[N]	[O]	[P]	[Q]	[R]	[S]	[T]
5	[A]	[B]	[C]	[D]	[E]	[F]	[G]	[H]	[I]	[J]	[K]	[L]	[M]	[N]	[O]	[P]	[Q]	[R]	[S]	[T]
6	[A]	[B]	[C]	[D]	[E]	[F]	[G]	[H]	[I]	[J]	[K]	[L]	[M]	[N]	[O]	[P]	[Q]	[R]	[S]	[T]
7	[A]	[B]	[C]	[D]	[E]	[F]	[G]	[H]	[I]	[J]	[K]	[L]	[M]	[N]	[O]	[P]	[Q]	[R]	[S]	[T]
8	[A]	[B]	[C]	[D]	[E]	[F]	[G]	[H]	[I]	[J]	[K]	[L]	[M]	[N]	[O]	[P]	[Q]	[R]	[S]	[T]
9	[A]	[B]	[C]	[D]	[E]	[F]	[G]	[H]	[I]	[J]	[K]	[L]	[M]	[N]	[O]	[P]	[Q]	[R]	[S]	[T]
10	[A]	[B]	[C]	[D]	[E]	[F]	[G]	[H]	[I]	[J]	[K]	[L]	[M]	[N]	[O]	[P]	[Q]	[R]	[S]	[T]
11	[A]	[B]	[C]	[D]	[E]	[F]	[G]	[H]	[I]	[J]	[K]	[L]	[M]	[N]	[O]	[P]	[Q]	[R]	[S]	[T]
12	[A]	[B]	[C]	[D]	[E]	[F]	[G]	[H]	[I]	[J]	[K]	[L]	[M]	[N]	[O]	[P]	[Q]	[R]	[S]	[T]
13	[A]	[B]	[C]	[D]	[E]	[F]	[G]	[H]	[I]	[J]	[K]	[L]	[M]	[N]	[O]	[P]	[Q]	[R]	[S]	[T]
14	[A]	[B]	[C]	[D]	[E]	[F]	[G]	[H]	[I]	[J]	[K]	[L]	[M]	[N]	[O]	[P]	[Q]	[R]	[S]	[T]
15	[A]	[B]	[C]	[D]	[E]	[F]	[G]	[H]	[I]	[J]	[K]	[L]	[M]	[N]	[O]	[P]	[Q]	[R]	[S]	[T]
16	[A]	[B]	[C]	[D]	[E]	[F]	[G]	[H]	[I]	[J]	[K]	[L]	[M]	[N]	[O]	[P]	[Q]	[R]	[S]	[T]
17	[A]	[B]	[C]	[D]	[E]	[F]	[G]	[H]	[I]	[J]	[K]	[L]	[M]	[N]	[O]	[P]	[Q]	[R]	[S]	[T]
18	[A]	[B]	[C]	[D]	[E]	[F]	[G]	[H]	[I]	[J]	[K]	[L]	[M]	[N]	[O]	[P]	[Q]	[R]	[S]	[T]
19	[A]	[B]	[C]	[D]	[E]	[F]	[G]	[H]	[I]	[J]	[K]	[L]	[M]	[N]	[O]	[P]	[Q]	[R]	[S]	[T]
20	[A]	[B]	[C]	[D]	[E]	[F]	[G]	[H]	[I]	[J]	[K]	[L]	[M]	[N]	[O]	[P]	[Q]	[R]	[S]	[T]

21	[A]	[B]	[C]	[D]	[E]	[F]	[G]	[H]	[I]	[J]	[K]	[L]	[M]	[N]	[O]	[P]	[Q]	[R]	[S]	[T]
22	[A]	[B]	[C]	[D]	[E]	[F]	[G]	[H]	[I]	[J]	[K]	[L]	[M]	[N]	[O]	[P]	[Q]	[R]	[S]	[T]
23	[A]	[B]	[C]	[D]	[E]	[F]	[G]	[H]	[I]	[J]	[K]	[L]	[M]	[N]	[O]	[P]	[Q]	[R]	[S]	[T]
24	[A]	[B]	[C]	[D]	[E]	[F]	[G]	[H]	[I]	[J]	[K]	[L]	[M]	[N]	[O]	[P]	[Q]	[R]	[S]	[T]
25	[A]	[B]	[C]	[D]	[E]	[F]	[G]	[H]	[I]	[J]	[K]	[L]	[M]	[N]	[O]	[P]	[Q]	[R]	[S]	[T]
26	[A]	[B]	[C]	[D]	[E]	[F]	[G]	[H]	[I]	[J]	[K]	[L]	[M]	[N]	[O]	[P]	[Q]	[R]	[S]	[T]
27	[A]	[B]	[C]	[D]	[E]	[F]	[G]	[H]	[I]	[J]	[K]	[L]	[M]	[N]	[O]	[P]	[Q]	[R]	[S]	[T]
28	[A]	[B]	[C]	[D]	[E]	[F]	[G]	[H]	[I]	[J]	[K]	[L]	[M]	[N]	[O]	[P]	[Q]	[R]	[S]	[T]
29	[A]	[B]	[C]	[D]	[E]	[F]	[G]	[H]	[I]	[J]	[K]	[L]	[M]	[N]	[O]	[P]	[Q]	[R]	[S]	[T]
20	[A]	[B]	[C]	[D]	[E]	[F]	[G]	[H]	[I]	[J]	[K]	[L]	[M]	[N]	[O]	[P]	[Q]	[R]	[S]	[T]
31	[A]	[B]	[C]	[D]	[E]	[F]	[G]	[H]	[I]	[J]	[K]	[L]	[M]	[N]	[O]	[P]	[Q]	[R]	[S]	[T]
32	[A]	[B]	[C]	[D]	[E]	[F]	[G]	[H]	[I]	[J]	[K]	[L]	[M]	[N]	[O]	[P]	[Q]	[R]	[S]	[T]
33	[A]	[B]	[C]	[D]	[E]	[F]	[G]	[H]	[I]	[J]	[K]	[L]	[M]	[N]	[O]	[P]	[Q]	[R]	[S]	[T]
34	[A]	[B]	[C]	[D]	[E]	[F]	[G]	[H]	[I]	[J]	[K]	[L]	[M]	[N]	[O]	[P]	[Q]	[R]	[S]	[T]
35	[A]	[B]	[C]	[D]	[E]	[F]	[G]	[H]	[I]	[J]	[K]	[L]	[M]	[N]	[O]	[P]	[Q]	[R]	[S]	[T]
36	[A]	[B]	[C]	[D]	[E]	[F]	[G]	[H]	[I]	[J]	[K]	[L]	[M]	[N]	[O]	[P]	[Q]	[R]	[S]	[T]
37	[A]	[B]	[C]	[D]	[E]	[F]	[G]	[H]	[I]	[J]	[K]	[L]	[M]	[N]	[O]	[P]	[Q]	[R]	[S]	[T]
38	[A]	[B]	[C]	[D]	[E]	[F]	[G]	[H]	[I]	[J]	[K]	[L]	[M]	[N]	[O]	[P]	[Q]	[R]	[S]	[T]
39	[A]	[B]	[C]	[D]	[E]	[F]	[G]	[H]	[I]	[J]	[K]	[L]	[M]	[N]	[O]	[P]	[Q]	[R]	[S]	[T]
40	[A]	[B]	[C]	[D]	[E]	[F]	[G]	[H]	[I]	[J]	[K]	[L]	[M]	[N]	[O]	[P]	[Q]	[R]	[S]	[T]

Mock examination answer sheet

Complete the sheet on the following page by fully filling in with pencil the lozenge corresponding to the **single** correct answer.

Please feel free to photocopy this sheet.

Index